LIVING WITH IBD AND CROHNS

A 6-Month Daily Companion for Your Healing Journey

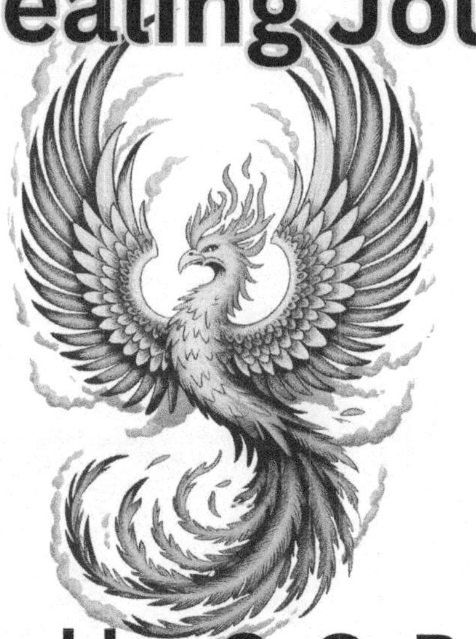

Created by C. G. Bromley

Copyright Info

Living With IBD and Crohns
Created by C. G. Bromley
Published by Jarlsberg Publishing
www.cristagoblebromley.com
First Edition

Who This Book is For

This tracking journal is for everyone who has ever felt unseen in their journey with Crohn's or IBD.

It is for the quiet fighters, the brave souls who carry on through pain, the ones who still notice small joys on hard days.

It is for you—because your story matters, your voice matters, and your daily steps deserve to be honored.

May these pages be a soft place to land.

From My Heart

"It took many years before I received my diagnosis of Crohn's disease. The road to get here was not easy—filled with confusing symptoms, trial after trial with medications, and the frustration of not being heard or understood. Through it all, I learned that healing is not just about the right medicine, but also about listening closely to my own body and caring for myself with patience and compassion. This journal grew out of my own need to keep track of food, energy, rest, feelings and much more—so I could see patterns that even doctors sometimes miss. My hope is that it helps you, too, not only to track your path, but also to move forward with resilience and a renewed sense of hope."

---C. G. Bromley

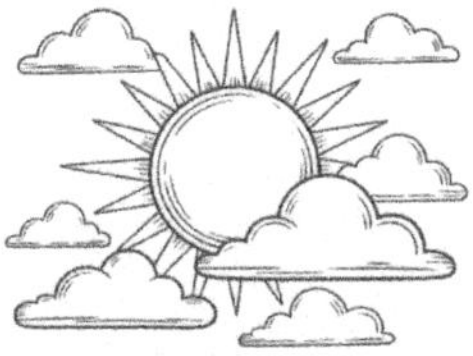

Welcome

This journal is your personal space to reflect, notice patterns, and capture the little details that often get lost in the day-to-day. Living with Crohn's or IBD can feel unpredictable, but writing things down can help you feel more grounded and prepared. Here, there are no right or wrong answers—just your story, in your own words. Use these pages to track meals, rest, energy, and feelings, but also to celebrate wins, jot down questions, and remind yourself of bright spots along the way. This is a tool for awareness and encouragement—not medical advice. Always follow the guidance of your healthcare team.
This journal is designed as a personal wellness and reflection tool for people living with Crohn's disease, IBD, or similar digestive challenges.

It is not a medical book and does not provide medical advice, diagnosis, or treatment. The information and prompts included here are for personal tracking and self-awareness only.

Always consult your doctor, specialist, or healthcare team for medical questions, treatment plans, or decisions about your health.

Every person's journey with Crohn's and IBD is unique. Use this journal as a supportive space to notice your own patterns, record your experiences, and reflect on your progress. If at any time you feel uncertain about your health or symptoms, please contact a qualified healthcare provider.

This is your story, your reflections, your journey.

Disclaimer

This journal is intended for personal reflection, organization, and encouragement. It is not a substitute for professional medical advice, diagnosis, or treatment. Always seek the advice of your physician or other qualified health provider with any questions you may have regarding a medical condition.

Do not disregard, avoid, or delay obtaining medical or health-related advice from your healthcare professional because of something you have read or tracked in this book.

The author and publisher make no representations or warranties about the completeness, reliability, or accuracy of the content. Use of this journal is voluntary and at your own discretion. The author and publisher are not responsible for any adverse effects, outcomes, or consequences resulting from the use of this book.

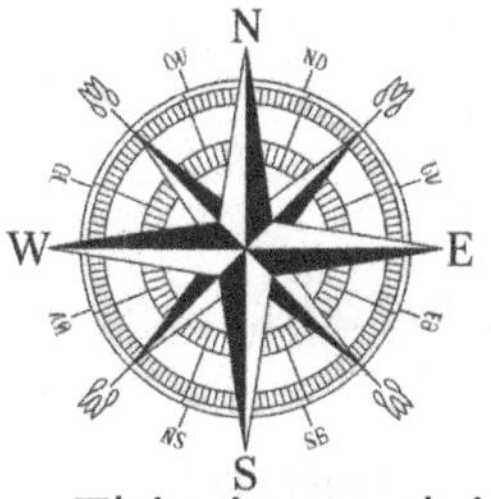

How To Use This Book

This journal is here to be your companion, not your homework. There are no rules, no grades, and no "perfect" way to fill it out. Think of it as a space that belongs completely to you, somewhere to capture the little details that matter most in your daily life with Crohn's or IBS.

What you'll find inside:

- Six-months of Daily Pages to track food, rest, energy, symptoms, and bright spots.
- Weekly Reflections to help you see patterns and think ahead.
- Monthly Overviews to step back and notice the bigger picture.
- Feelings Pages to give space for your emotions and mental well-being.
- Doctor Notes to keep important updates and instructions in one place.
- Questions for Doctors so you remember what matters most during visits.
- Hospital log
- Medication & Treatment Logs
- Steroid tracking chart, and MORE

Sometimes your emotions may need a place of their own. In the back of this journal, you'll find a page created for different moods. If you're feeling one of these, flip to that section for a gentle word, a prompt, or a space to reflect:

- Anxious
- Discouraged
- Overwhelmed
- Hopeful
- Grateful
- Content

A few gentle suggestions:

- Start with today. Don't worry about "catching up." Each page is a fresh start.
- Be honest, not perfect. Write what really happened, even if it feels small or messy.
- Notice patterns, not judgments. This is about awareness, not blame. A tough day is just a page, not your whole story.
- Celebrate wins. Even tiny victories, like a meal that sat well, or a moment you laughed, deserve to be written down.
- Make it yours. Use doodles, stickers, color coding, or notes in the margins. This is your safe space.

Remember, this journal is a tool for you. Skip sections when you need to, write more when you want to, and never feel pressured to fill in every line.

Your journey isn't defined by symptoms—it's shaped by resilience, growth, and hope. Let this journal be a gentle witness along the way.

Daily Tracking

DATE:

S M T W T F S

Meal Tracking

Fluid Tracker: 8 oz | 8 oz | 8 oz | 8 oz | 8 oz | 8 oz | 8 oz | 8 oz

Time	Meal	Pain Scale 0-5 0= No pain 5= Severe
BREAKFAST		
LUNCH		
DINNER		
SNACKS		

Bowel Activity

Normal	Very Hard	Abnormalities
		☐ Blood ☐ Mucus ☐ Other ______
		☐ Blood ☐ Mucus ☐ Other ______
		☐ Blood ☐ Mucus ☐ Other ______
		☐ Blood ☐ Mucus ☐ Other ______
	More?	

Other Symptoms

- ☐ Bloating
- ☐ Fatigue
- ☐ Nausea
- ☐ Flatulence
- ☐ Vomiting
- ☐ Other ______________________

Stress Level

Sleep

Energy Level

Activity Level

Pain Location (If Applicable)

- ☐ Abdomen
- ☐ Joints
- ☐ Stomach
- ☐ Rectum
- ☐ Other ______________________

Medications

____

____

____

____

____

Notes

Daily Tracking

DATE:

S M T W T F S

Fluid Tracker: 8 oz | 8 oz | 8 oz | 8 oz | 8 oz | 8 oz | 8 oz | 8 oz

Meal Tracking

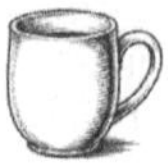

Time	Meal	Pain Scale 0-5 0= No pain 5= Severe
BREAKFAST		
LUNCH		
DINNER		
SNACKS		

Bowel Activity

Normal	Very Hard	Abnormalities
		☐ Blood ☐ Mucus ☐ Other ______
		☐ Blood ☐ Mucus ☐ Other ______
		☐ Blood ☐ Mucus ☐ Other ______
		☐ Blood ☐ Mucus ☐ Other ______
	More?	

Other Symptoms

☐ Bloating ☐ Fatigue
☐ Nausea ☐ Flatulence
☐ Vomiting
☐ Other ______________________

Stress Level

Sleep

Energy Level

Activity Level

Pain Location (If Applicable)

☐ Abdomen ☐ Joints
☐ Stomach ☐ Rectum
☐ Other ______________________

Medications

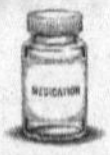

____
____
____
____
____

Notes

Daily Tracking

DATE:

S M T W T F S

Fluid Tracker 8 oz 8 oz 8 oz 8 oz 8 oz 8 oz 8 oz 8 oz

Meal Tracking

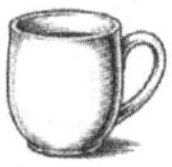

Time	Meal	Pain Scale 0-5 0= No pain 5= Severe
BREAKFAST		
LUNCH		
DINNER		
SNACKS		

Bowel Activity

Normal	Very Hard	Abnormalities
		☐ Blood ☐ Mucus ☐ Other ______
		☐ Blood ☐ Mucus ☐ Other ______
		☐ Blood ☐ Mucus ☐ Other ______
		☐ Blood ☐ Mucus ☐ Other ______
	More?	

Other Symptoms

☐ Bloating ☐ Fatigue
☐ Nausea ☐ Flatulence
☐ Vomiting
☐ Other ______________________

Stress Level

Sleep

Energy Level

Activity Level

Pain Location (If Applicable)

☐ Abdomen ☐ Joints
☐ Stomach ☐ Rectum
☐ Other ______________________

Notes

Medications

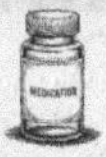

____

____

____

____

____

Daily Tracking

DATE:

S M T W T F S

Fluid Tracker: 8 oz | 8 oz | 8 oz | 8 oz | 8 oz | 8 oz | 8 oz | 8 oz

Meal Tracking

Time	Meal	Pain Scale 0-5 0= No pain 5= Severe
BREAKFAST		
LUNCH		
DINNER		
SNACKS		

Bowel Activity

Normal	Very Hard	Abnormalities
		☐ Blood ☐ Mucus ☐ Other ______
		☐ Blood ☐ Mucus ☐ Other ______
		☐ Blood ☐ Mucus ☐ Other ______
		☐ Blood ☐ Mucus ☐ Other ______
	More?	

Other Symptoms

☐ Bloating ☐ Fatigue
☐ Nausea ☐ Flatulence
☐ Vomiting
☐ Other ____________________

Stress Level

Sleep

Energy Level

Activity Level

Pain Location (If Applicable)

☐ Abdomen ☐ Joints
☐ Stomach ☐ Rectum
☐ Other ____________________

Medications

____
____
____
____
____

Notes

Daily Tracking

DATE:

S M T W T F S

Fluid Tracker: 8 oz | 8 oz | 8 oz | 8 oz | 8 oz | 8 oz | 8 oz | 8 oz

Meal Tracking

Time	Meal	Pain Scale 0-5 0= No pain 5= Severe
BREAKFAST		
LUNCH		
DINNER		
SNACKS		

Bowel Activity

Normal	Very Hard	Abnormalities
		☐ Blood ☐ Mucus ☐ Other ______
		☐ Blood ☐ Mucus ☐ Other ______
		☐ Blood ☐ Mucus ☐ Other ______
		☐ Blood ☐ Mucus ☐ Other ______
	More?	

Other Symptoms

☐ Bloating ☐ Fatigue
☐ Nausea ☐ Flatulence
☐ Vomiting
☐ Other ______________________

Stress Level

Sleep

Energy Level

Activity Level

Pain Location (If Applicable)

☐ Abdomen ☐ Joints
☐ Stomach ☐ Rectum
☐ Other ______________________

Medications

____
____
____
____
____

Notes

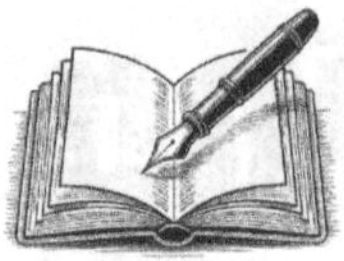

Daily Tracking

DATE:

S M T W T F S

Fluid Tracker 8 oz 8 oz 8 oz 8 oz 8 oz 8 oz 8 oz 8 oz

Meal Tracking

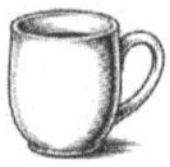

Time	Meal	Pain Scale 0-5 0= No pain 5= Severe
BREAKFAST		
LUNCH		
DINNER		
SNACKS		

Bowel Activity

Normal	Very Hard	Abnormalities
		☐ Blood ☐ Mucus ☐ Other ______
		☐ Blood ☐ Mucus ☐ Other ______
		☐ Blood ☐ Mucus ☐ Other ______
		☐ Blood ☐ Mucus ☐ Other ______
	More?	

Other Symptoms

- ☐ Bloating
- ☐ Fatigue
- ☐ Nausea
- ☐ Flatulence
- ☐ Vomiting
- ☐ Other ______________________

Stress Level

Sleep

Energy Level

Activity Level

Pain Location (If Applicable)

- ☐ Abdomen
- ☐ Joints
- ☐ Stomach
- ☐ Rectum
- ☐ Other ______________________

Notes

Medications

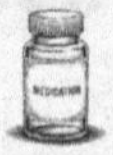

____

____

____

____

____

Daily Tracking

DATE:

S M T W T F S

Fluid Tracker: 8 oz | 8 oz | 8 oz | 8 oz | 8 oz | 8 oz | 8 oz | 8 oz

Meal Tracking

Time	Meal	Pain Scale 0-5 0= No pain 5= Severe
BREAKFAST		
LUNCH		
DINNER		
SNACKS		

Bowel Activity

Normal	Very Hard	Abnormalities
		☐ Blood ☐ Mucus ☐ Other ______
		☐ Blood ☐ Mucus ☐ Other ______
		☐ Blood ☐ Mucus ☐ Other ______
		☐ Blood ☐ Mucus ☐ Other ______
	More?	

Other Symptoms

☐ Bloating ☐ Fatigue
☐ Nausea ☐ Flatulence
☐ Vomiting
☐ Other ______

Stress Level

Sleep

Energy Level

Activity Level

Pain Location (If Applicable)

☐ Abdomen ☐ Joints
☐ Stomach ☐ Rectum
☐ Other ______

Medications

______
______
______
______
______

Notes

Weekly Reflections

What was the best thing that happened this week?

What was the hardest thing that happened this week?

What helped you the most this week?

What gave you hope this week?

What's one small win you can celebrate?

Was there something that eased your stress?

Overall, this week I felt

☐ A little better ☐ A lot better ☐ A little worse ☐ A lot worse
☐ About the same

Next week I want to:

____

____

____

____

'Every step you take toward listening to your body matters. Small notes today may become powerful insights tomorrow.'

Daily Tracking

DATE:

S M T W T F S

Fluid Tracker: 8 oz | 8 oz | 8 oz | 8 oz | 8 oz | 8 oz | 8 oz | 8 oz

Meal Tracking

Time	Meal	Pain Scale 0-5 0= No pain 5= Severe
BREAKFAST		
LUNCH		
DINNER		
SNACKS		

Bowel Activity

Normal	Very Hard	Abnormalities
		☐ Blood ☐ Mucus ☐ Other ______
		☐ Blood ☐ Mucus ☐ Other ______
		☐ Blood ☐ Mucus ☐ Other ______
		☐ Blood ☐ Mucus ☐ Other ______
	More?	

Other Symptoms

☐ Bloating ☐ Fatigue
☐ Nausea ☐ Flatulence
☐ Vomiting
☐ Other ______

Stress Level

Sleep

Energy Level

Activity Level

Pain Location (If Applicable)

☐ Abdomen ☐ Joints
☐ Stomach ☐ Rectum
☐ Other ______

Medications

______
______
______
______
______

Notes

Daily Tracking

DATE:

S M T W T F S

Fluid Tracker: 8 oz | 8 oz | 8 oz | 8 oz | 8 oz | 8 oz | 8 oz | 8 oz

Meal Tracking

Time	Meal	Pain Scale 0-5 0= No pain 5= Severe
BREAKFAST		
LUNCH		
DINNER		
SNACKS		

Bowel Activity

Normal	Very Hard	Abnormalities
		☐ Blood ☐ Mucus ☐ Other ______
		☐ Blood ☐ Mucus ☐ Other ______
		☐ Blood ☐ Mucus ☐ Other ______
		☐ Blood ☐ Mucus ☐ Other ______
	More?	

Other Symptoms

☐ Bloating ☐ Fatigue
☐ Nausea ☐ Flatulence
☐ Vomiting
☐ Other ______________________

Stress Level

Sleep

Energy Level

Activity Level

Pain Location (If Applicable)

☐ Abdomen ☐ Joints
☐ Stomach ☐ Rectum
☐ Other ______________________

Medications

____
____
____
____
____

Notes

Daily Tracking

DATE:

S M T W T F S

Fluid Tracker: 8 oz | 8 oz | 8 oz | 8 oz | 8 oz | 8 oz | 8 oz | 8 oz

Meal Tracking

Time	Meal	Pain Scale 0-5 0= No pain 5= Severe
BREAKFAST		
LUNCH		
DINNER		
SNACKS		

Bowel Activity

Normal	Very Hard	Abnormalities
		☐ Blood ☐ Mucus ☐ Other ______
		☐ Blood ☐ Mucus ☐ Other ______
		☐ Blood ☐ Mucus ☐ Other ______
		☐ Blood ☐ Mucus ☐ Other ______
	More?	

Other Symptoms

- ☐ Bloating
- ☐ Fatigue
- ☐ Nausea
- ☐ Flatulence
- ☐ Vomiting
- ☐ Other ______________________

Stress Level

Sleep

Energy Level

Activity Level

Pain Location (If Applicable)

- ☐ Abdomen
- ☐ Joints
- ☐ Stomach
- ☐ Rectum
- ☐ Other ______________________

Medications

____

____

____

____

____

Notes

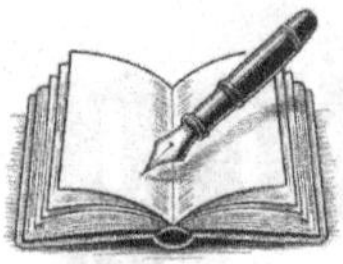

Daily Tracking

DATE:

S M T W T F S

Fluid Tracker: 8 oz | 8 oz | 8 oz | 8 oz | 8 oz | 8 oz | 8 oz | 8 oz

Meal Tracking

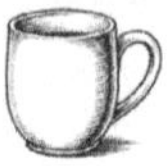

Time	Meal	Pain Scale 0-5 0= No pain 5= Severe
BREAKFAST		
LUNCH		
DINNER		
SNACKS		

Bowel Activity

Normal	Very Hard	Abnormalities
		☐ Blood ☐ Mucus ☐ Other ______
		☐ Blood ☐ Mucus ☐ Other ______
		☐ Blood ☐ Mucus ☐ Other ______
		☐ Blood ☐ Mucus ☐ Other ______
	More?	

Other Symptoms

☐ Bloating ☐ Fatigue

☐ Nausea ☐ Flatulence

☐ Vomiting

☐ Other ______________________

Stress Level

Sleep

Energy Level

Activity Level

Pain Location (If Applicable)

☐ Abdomen ☐ Joints

☐ Stomach ☐ Rectum

☐ Other ______________________

Notes

Medications

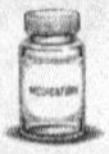

____

____

____

____

____

Daily Tracking

DATE:

S M T W T F S

Fluid Tracker: 8 oz | 8 oz | 8 oz | 8 oz | 8 oz | 8 oz | 8 oz | 8 oz

Meal Tracking

Time	Meal	Pain Scale 0-5 0= No pain 5= Severe
BREAKFAST		
LUNCH		
DINNER		
SNACKS		

Bowel Activity

Normal	Very Hard	Abnormalities
		☐ Blood ☐ Mucus ☐ Other ______
		☐ Blood ☐ Mucus ☐ Other ______
		☐ Blood ☐ Mucus ☐ Other ______
		☐ Blood ☐ Mucus ☐ Other ______
	More?	

Other Symptoms

- ☐ Bloating
- ☐ Fatigue
- ☐ Nausea
- ☐ Flatulence
- ☐ Vomiting
- ☐ Other ______________________

Stress Level

Sleep

Energy Level

Activity Level

Pain Location (If Applicable)

- ☐ Abdomen
- ☐ Joints
- ☐ Stomach
- ☐ Rectum
- ☐ Other ______________________

Medications

____

____

____

____

____

Notes

Daily Tracking

DATE:

S M T W T F S

Fluid Tracker 8 oz 8 oz 8 oz 8 oz 8 oz 8 oz 8 oz 8 oz

Meal Tracking

Time	Meal	Pain Scale 0-5 0= No pain 5= Severe
BREAKFAST		
LUNCH		
DINNER		
SNACKS		

Bowel Activity

Normal	Very Hard	Abnormalities
		☐ Blood ☐ Mucus ☐ Other ______
		☐ Blood ☐ Mucus ☐ Other ______
		☐ Blood ☐ Mucus ☐ Other ______
		☐ Blood ☐ Mucus ☐ Other ______
	More?	

Other Symptoms

☐ Bloating ☐ Fatigue
☐ Nausea ☐ Flatulence
☐ Vomiting
☐ Other ______________________

Stress Level

Sleep

Energy Level

Activity Level

Pain Location (If Applicable)

☐ Abdomen ☐ Joints
☐ Stomach ☐ Rectum
☐ Other ______________________

Notes

Medications

____
____
____
____
____

Daily Tracking

DATE:

S M T W T F S

Meal Tracking

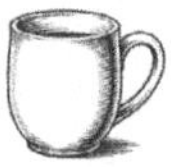

Fluid Tracker: 8 oz | 8 oz | 8 oz | 8 oz | 8 oz | 8 oz | 8 oz | 8 oz

Time	Meal	Pain Scale 0-5 0= No pain 5= Severe
BREAKFAST		
LUNCH		
DINNER		
SNACKS		

Bowel Activity

Normal	Very Hard	Abnormalities
		☐ Blood ☐ Mucus ☐ Other ____
		☐ Blood ☐ Mucus ☐ Other ____
		☐ Blood ☐ Mucus ☐ Other ____
		☐ Blood ☐ Mucus ☐ Other ____
	More?	

Other Symptoms

☐ Bloating ☐ Fatigue
☐ Nausea ☐ Flatulence
☐ Vomiting
☐ Other ____________________

Stress Level

Sleep

Energy Level

Activity Level

Pain Location (If Applicable)

☐ Abdomen ☐ Joints
☐ Stomach ☐ Rectum
☐ Other ____________________

Medications

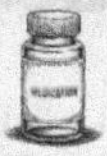

____
____
____
____
____

Notes

Daily Tracking

DATE:

S M T W T F S

Fluid Tracker: 8 oz | 8 oz | 8 oz | 8 oz | 8 oz | 8 oz | 8 oz | 8 oz

Meal Tracking

Time	Meal	Pain Scale 0-5 0= No pain 5= Severe
BREAKFAST		
LUNCH		
DINNER		
SNACKS		

Bowel Activity

Normal	Very Hard	Abnormalities
		☐ Blood ☐ Mucus ☐ Other ______
		☐ Blood ☐ Mucus ☐ Other ______
		☐ Blood ☐ Mucus ☐ Other ______
		☐ Blood ☐ Mucus ☐ Other ______
	More?	

Other Symptoms

☐ Bloating ☐ Fatigue
☐ Nausea ☐ Flatulence
☐ Vomiting
☐ Other ______________________

Stress Level

Sleep

Energy Level

Activity Level

Pain Location (If Applicable)

☐ Abdomen ☐ Joints
☐ Stomach ☐ Rectum
☐ Other ______________________

Medications

____
____
____
____
____

Notes

Weekly Reflections

What was the best thing that happened this week?

What was the hardest thing that happened this week?

What helped you the most this week?

What gave you hope this week?

What's one small win you can celebrate?

Was there something that eased your stress?

Overall, this week I felt

☐ A little better ☐ A lot better ☐ A little worse ☐ A lot worse

☐ About the same

Next week I want to:

____

____

____

____

Healing is not a straight line. Give yourself permission to rest when you need to.

Daily Tracking

DATE:

S M T W T F S

Fluid Tracker: 8 oz 8 oz 8 oz 8 oz 8 oz 8 oz 8 oz 8 oz

Meal Tracking

Time	Meal	Pain Scale 0-5 0= No pain 5= Severe
BREAKFAST		
LUNCH		
DINNER		
SNACKS		

Bowel Activity

Normal	Very Hard	Abnormalities
		☐ Blood ☐ Mucus ☐ Other ______
		☐ Blood ☐ Mucus ☐ Other ______
		☐ Blood ☐ Mucus ☐ Other ______
		☐ Blood ☐ Mucus ☐ Other ______
	More?	

Other Symptoms

☐ Bloating ☐ Fatigue
☐ Nausea ☐ Flatulence
☐ Vomiting
☐ Other ______________________

Stress Level

Sleep

Energy Level

Activity Level

Pain Location (If Applicable)

☐ Abdomen ☐ Joints
☐ Stomach ☐ Rectum
☐ Other ______________________

Medications

____
____
____
____
____

Notes

Daily Tracking

DATE:

S M T W T F S

Fluid Tracker: 8 oz 8 oz 8 oz 8 oz 8 oz 8 oz 8 oz 8 oz

Meal Tracking

Time	Meal	Pain Scale 0-5 0= No pain 5= Severe
BREAKFAST		
LUNCH		
DINNER		
SNACKS		

Bowel Activity

Normal	Very Hard	Abnormalities
		☐ Blood ☐ Mucus ☐ Other ______
		☐ Blood ☐ Mucus ☐ Other ______
		☐ Blood ☐ Mucus ☐ Other ______
		☐ Blood ☐ Mucus ☐ Other ______
	More?	

Other Symptoms

☐ Bloating ☐ Fatigue
☐ Nausea ☐ Flatulence
☐ Vomiting
☐ Other ______________________

Stress Level

Sleep

Energy Level

Activity Level

Pain Location (If Applicable)

☐ Abdomen ☐ Joints
☐ Stomach ☐ Rectum
☐ Other ______________________

Medications

____
____
____
____
____

Notes

Daily Tracking

DATE:

S M T W T F S

Meal Tracking

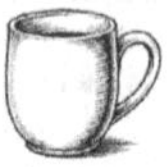

Fluid Tracker: 8 oz | 8 oz | 8 oz | 8 oz | 8 oz | 8 oz | 8 oz | 8 oz

Time	Meal	Pain Scale 0-5 0= No pain 5= Severe
BREAKFAST		
LUNCH		
DINNER		
SNACKS		

Bowel Activity

Normal	Very Hard	Abnormalities
		☐ Blood ☐ Mucus ☐ Other ______
		☐ Blood ☐ Mucus ☐ Other ______
		☐ Blood ☐ Mucus ☐ Other ______
		☐ Blood ☐ Mucus ☐ Other ______
	More?	

Other Symptoms

☐ Bloating ☐ Fatigue
☐ Nausea ☐ Flatulence
☐ Vomiting
☐ Other ______________________

Stress Level

Sleep

Energy Level

Activity Level

Pain Location (If Applicable)

☐ Abdomen ☐ Joints
☐ Stomach ☐ Rectum
☐ Other ______________________

Medications

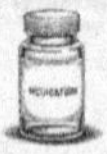

____
____
____
____
____

Notes

Daily Tracking

DATE:

S M T W T F S

Fluid Tracker: 8 oz | 8 oz | 8 oz | 8 oz | 8 oz | 8 oz | 8 oz | 8 oz

Meal Tracking

Time	Meal	Pain Scale 0-5 0= No pain 5= Severe
BREAKFAST		
LUNCH		
DINNER		
SNACKS		

Bowel Activity

Normal	Very Hard	Abnormalities
		☐ Blood ☐ Mucus ☐ Other ______
		☐ Blood ☐ Mucus ☐ Other ______
		☐ Blood ☐ Mucus ☐ Other ______
		☐ Blood ☐ Mucus ☐ Other ______
	More?	

Other Symptoms

☐ Bloating ☐ Fatigue
☐ Nausea ☐ Flatulence
☐ Vomiting
☐ Other ______________________

Stress Level

Sleep

Energy Level

Activity Level

Pain Location (If Applicable)

☐ Abdomen ☐ Joints
☐ Stomach ☐ Rectum
☐ Other ______________________

Medications

____
____
____
____
____

Notes

Daily Tracking

DATE:

S M T W T F S

Fluid Tracker: 8 oz | 8 oz | 8 oz | 8 oz | 8 oz | 8 oz | 8 oz | 8 oz

Meal Tracking

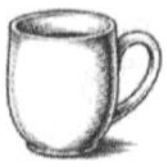

Time	Meal	Pain Scale 0-5 0= No pain 5= Severe
BREAKFAST		
LUNCH		
DINNER		
SNACKS		

Bowel Activity

Normal	Very Hard	Abnormalities
		☐ Blood ☐ Mucus ☐ Other ______
		☐ Blood ☐ Mucus ☐ Other ______
		☐ Blood ☐ Mucus ☐ Other ______
		☐ Blood ☐ Mucus ☐ Other ______
	More?	

Other Symptoms

☐ Bloating ☐ Fatigue
☐ Nausea ☐ Flatulence
☐ Vomiting
☐ Other ______________________

Stress Level

Sleep

Energy Level

Activity Level

Pain Location (If Applicable)

☐ Abdomen ☐ Joints
☐ Stomach ☐ Rectum
☐ Other ______________________

Notes

Medications

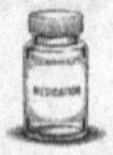

____

____

____

____

____

Daily Tracking

DATE:

S M T W T F S

Fluid Tracker: 8 oz | 8 oz | 8 oz | 8 oz | 8 oz | 8 oz | 8 oz | 8 oz

Meal Tracking

Time	Meal	Pain Scale 0-5 0= No pain 5= Severe
BREAKFAST		
LUNCH		
DINNER		
SNACKS		

Bowel Activity

Normal	Very Hard	Abnormalities
		☐ Blood ☐ Mucus ☐ Other ______
		☐ Blood ☐ Mucus ☐ Other ______
		☐ Blood ☐ Mucus ☐ Other ______
		☐ Blood ☐ Mucus ☐ Other ______
	More?	

Other Symptoms

☐ Bloating ☐ Fatigue
☐ Nausea ☐ Flatulence
☐ Vomiting
☐ Other ______________________

Stress Level

Sleep

Energy Level

Activity Level

Pain Location (If Applicable)

☐ Abdomen ☐ Joints
☐ Stomach ☐ Rectum
☐ Other ______________________

Medications

____
____
____
____
____

Notes

Daily Tracking

DATE:

S M T W T F S

Fluid Tracker: 8 oz 8 oz 8 oz 8 oz 8 oz 8 oz 8 oz 8 oz

Meal Tracking

Time	Meal	Pain Scale 0-5 0= No pain 5= Severe
BREAKFAST		
LUNCH		
DINNER		
SNACKS		

Bowel Activity

Normal	Very Hard	Abnormalities
		☐ Blood ☐ Mucus ☐ Other ______
		☐ Blood ☐ Mucus ☐ Other ______
		☐ Blood ☐ Mucus ☐ Other ______
		☐ Blood ☐ Mucus ☐ Other ______
	More?	

Other Symptoms

☐ Bloating ☐ Fatigue
☐ Nausea ☐ Flatulence
☐ Vomiting
☐ Other ______________________

Stress Level

Sleep

Energy Level

Activity Level

Pain Location (If Applicable)

☐ Abdomen ☐ Joints
☐ Stomach ☐ Rectum
☐ Other ______________________

Notes

Medications

____
____
____
____
____

Weekly Reflections

What was the best thing that happened this week?

What was the hardest thing that happened this week?

What helped you the most this week?

What gave you hope this week?

What's one small win you can celebrate?

Was there something that eased your stress?

Overall, this week I felt

☐ A little better ☐ A lot better ☐ A little worse ☐ A lot worse

☐ About the same

Next week I want to:

____

____

____

____

Even in hard weeks, there are bright moments worth holding onto. Look for one spark each day.

Daily Tracking

DATE:

S M T W T F S

Fluid Tracker: 8 oz | 8 oz | 8 oz | 8 oz | 8 oz | 8 oz | 8 oz | 8 oz

Meal Tracking

Time	Meal	Pain Scale 0-5 0= No pain 5= Severe
BREAKFAST		
LUNCH		
DINNER		
SNACKS		

Bowel Activity

Normal	Very Hard	Abnormalities
		☐ Blood ☐ Mucus ☐ Other ______
		☐ Blood ☐ Mucus ☐ Other ______
		☐ Blood ☐ Mucus ☐ Other ______
		☐ Blood ☐ Mucus ☐ Other ______
	More?	

Other Symptoms

☐ Bloating ☐ Fatigue
☐ Nausea ☐ Flatulence
☐ Vomiting
☐ Other ____________________

Stress Level

Sleep

Energy Level

Activity Level

Pain Location (If Applicable)

☐ Abdomen ☐ Joints
☐ Stomach ☐ Rectum
☐ Other ____________________

Medications

____
____
____
____
____

Notes

Daily Tracking

DATE:

S M T W T F S

Fluid Tracker: 8 oz | 8 oz | 8 oz | 8 oz | 8 oz | 8 oz | 8 oz | 8 oz

Meal Tracking

Time	Meal	Pain Scale 0-5 0= No pain 5= Severe
BREAKFAST		
LUNCH		
DINNER		
SNACKS		

Bowel Activity

Normal	Very Hard	Abnormalities
		☐ Blood ☐ Mucus ☐ Other ______
		☐ Blood ☐ Mucus ☐ Other ______
		☐ Blood ☐ Mucus ☐ Other ______
		☐ Blood ☐ Mucus ☐ Other ______
	More?	

Other Symptoms

- ☐ Bloating
- ☐ Fatigue
- ☐ Nausea
- ☐ Flatulence
- ☐ Vomiting
- ☐ Other ______________________

Stress Level

Sleep

Energy Level

Activity Level

Pain Location (If Applicable)

- ☐ Abdomen
- ☐ Joints
- ☐ Stomach
- ☐ Rectum
- ☐ Other ______________________

Notes

Medications

____

____

____

____

____

Daily Tracking

DATE: | S M T W T F S

Meal Tracking

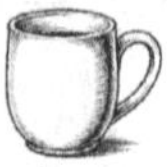

Fluid Tracker 8 oz 8 oz 8 oz 8 oz 8 oz 8 oz 8 oz 8 oz

Time	Meal	Pain Scale 0-5 0= No pain 5= Severe
BREAKFAST		
LUNCH		
DINNER		
SNACKS		

Bowel Activity

Normal	Very Hard	Abnormalities
		☐ Blood ☐ Mucus ☐ Other ______
		☐ Blood ☐ Mucus ☐ Other ______
		☐ Blood ☐ Mucus ☐ Other ______
		☐ Blood ☐ Mucus ☐ Other ______
	More?	

Other Symptoms

☐ Bloating ☐ Fatigue
☐ Nausea ☐ Flatulence
☐ Vomiting
☐ Other ______________________

Stress Level

Sleep

Energy Level

Activity Level

Pain Location (If Applicable)

☐ Abdomen ☐ Joints
☐ Stomach ☐ Rectum
☐ Other ______________________

Medications

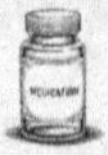

____
____
____
____
____

Notes

Daily Tracking

DATE:

S M T W T F S

Meal Tracking

Fluid Tracker: 8 oz | 8 oz | 8 oz | 8 oz | 8 oz | 8 oz | 8 oz | 8 oz

Time	Meal	Pain Scale 0-5 0= No pain 5= Severe
BREAKFAST		
LUNCH		
DINNER		
SNACKS		

Bowel Activity

Normal	Very Hard	Abnormalities
		☐ Blood ☐ Mucus ☐ Other
		☐ Blood ☐ Mucus ☐ Other
		☐ Blood ☐ Mucus ☐ Other
		☐ Blood ☐ Mucus ☐ Other
	More?	

Other Symptoms

☐ Bloating ☐ Fatigue
☐ Nausea ☐ Flatulence
☐ Vomiting
☐ Other

Stress Level

Sleep

Energy Level

Activity Level

Pain Location (If Applicable)

☐ Abdomen ☐ Joints
☐ Stomach ☐ Rectum
☐ Other

Medications

Notes

Daily Tracking

DATE:

S M T W T F S

Fluid Tracker 8 oz 8 oz 8 oz 8 oz 8 oz 8 oz 8 oz 8 oz

Meal Tracking

Time	Meal	Pain Scale 0-5 0= No pain 5= Severe
BREAKFAST		
LUNCH		
DINNER		
SNACKS		

Bowel Activity

Normal	Very Hard	Abnormalities
		☐ Blood ☐ Mucus ☐ Other ______
		☐ Blood ☐ Mucus ☐ Other ______
		☐ Blood ☐ Mucus ☐ Other ______
		☐ Blood ☐ Mucus ☐ Other ______
	More?	

Other Symptoms

☐ Bloating ☐ Fatigue
☐ Nausea ☐ Flatulence
☐ Vomiting
☐ Other ______

Stress Level

Sleep

Energy Level

Activity Level

Pain Location (If Applicable)

☐ Abdomen ☐ Joints
☐ Stomach ☐ Rectum
☐ Other ______

Medications

Notes

Daily Tracking

DATE:

S M T W T F S

Fluid Tracker: 8 oz | 8 oz | 8 oz | 8 oz | 8 oz | 8 oz | 8 oz | 8 oz

Meal Tracking

Time	Meal	Pain Scale 0-5 0= No pain 5= Severe
BREAKFAST		
LUNCH		
DINNER		
SNACKS		

Bowel Activity

Normal	Very Hard	Abnormalities
		☐ Blood ☐ Mucus ☐ Other ____
		☐ Blood ☐ Mucus ☐ Other ____
		☐ Blood ☐ Mucus ☐ Other ____
		☐ Blood ☐ Mucus ☐ Other ____
	More?	

Other Symptoms

☐ Bloating ☐ Fatigue
☐ Nausea ☐ Flatulence
☐ Vomiting
☐ Other ____________________

Stress Level

Sleep

Energy Level

Activity Level

Pain Location (If Applicable)

☐ Abdomen ☐ Joints
☐ Stomach ☐ Rectum
☐ Other ____________________

Medications

____
____
____
____
____

Notes

Daily Tracking

DATE:

S M T W T F S

Fluid Tracker: 8 oz | 8 oz | 8 oz | 8 oz | 8 oz | 8 oz | 8 oz | 8 oz

Meal Tracking

Time	Meal	Pain Scale 0-5 0= No pain 5= Severe
BREAKFAST		
LUNCH		
DINNER		
SNACKS		

Bowel Activity

Normal	Very Hard	Abnormalities
		☐ Blood ☐ Mucus ☐ Other ____
		☐ Blood ☐ Mucus ☐ Other ____
		☐ Blood ☐ Mucus ☐ Other ____
		☐ Blood ☐ Mucus ☐ Other ____
	More?	

Other Symptoms

☐ Bloating ☐ Fatigue
☐ Nausea ☐ Flatulence
☐ Vomiting
☐ Other ____________________

Stress Level

Sleep

Energy Level

Activity Level

Pain Location (If Applicable)

☐ Abdomen ☐ Joints
☐ Stomach ☐ Rectum
☐ Other ____________________

Medications

____
____
____
____
____

Notes

Weekly Reflections

What was the best thing that happened this week?

What was the hardest thing that happened this week?

What helped you the most this week?

What gave you hope this week?

What's one small win you can celebrate?

Was there something that eased your stress?

Overall, this week I felt

☐ A little better ☐ A lot better ☐ A little worse ☐ A lot worse

☐ About the same

Next week I want to:

____

____

____

____

IMPORTANT REMINDER

Your body is unique, and so is your path. Trust that learning your patterns is a form of self-care.

Monthly Thoughts

This page is your space to step back and see the bigger picture. Each month brings its own challenges and small victories—use this space to notice patterns, celebrate progress, and reflect on what your body and mind are teaching you. These notes can guide you forward with greater clarity and self-compassion.

This Month I Noticed...

(Write down patterns in your symptoms, energy, or mood.)

Biggest Challenge: ____

____

Brightest Moment: ____

____

Triggers I Noticed: ____

____

Things That Helped: ____

____

Medication / Treatment Notes: (Any changes, side effects, or adjustments.) ____

____

____

Self-Care Check-In

How well I cared for myself this month: ______________________

____

Looking Forward

Next month I want to focus on: ______________________

____

____

Symptom Overview

Good Days: ________ Mild Days: ________ Flare Days: ________

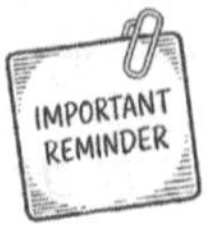

Beginnings don't have to be big—they just need to be honest.

Daily Tracking

DATE:

S M T W T F S

Fluid Tracker: 8 oz | 8 oz | 8 oz | 8 oz | 8 oz | 8 oz | 8 oz | 8 oz

Meal Tracking

Time	Meal	Pain Scale 0-5 0= No pain 5= Severe
BREAKFAST		
LUNCH		
DINNER		
SNACKS		

Bowel Activity

Normal	Very Hard	Abnormalities
		☐ Blood ☐ Mucus ☐ Other ______
		☐ Blood ☐ Mucus ☐ Other ______
		☐ Blood ☐ Mucus ☐ Other ______
		☐ Blood ☐ Mucus ☐ Other ______
	More?	

Other Symptoms

☐ Bloating ☐ Fatigue
☐ Nausea ☐ Flatulence
☐ Vomiting
☐ Other ______

Stress Level

Sleep

Energy Level

Activity Level

Pain Location (If Applicable)

☐ Abdomen ☐ Joints
☐ Stomach ☐ Rectum
☐ Other ______

Medications

______
______
______
______
______

Notes

Daily Tracking

DATE:

S M T W T F S

Meal Tracking

Fluid Tracker: 8 oz | 8 oz | 8 oz | 8 oz | 8 oz | 8 oz | 8 oz | 8 oz

Time	Meal	Pain Scale 0-5 0= No pain 5= Severe
BREAKFAST		
LUNCH		
DINNER		
SNACKS		

Bowel Activity

Normal	Very Hard	Abnormalities
		☐ Blood ☐ Mucus ☐ Other ______
		☐ Blood ☐ Mucus ☐ Other ______
		☐ Blood ☐ Mucus ☐ Other ______
		☐ Blood ☐ Mucus ☐ Other ______
	More?	

Pain Location (If Applicable)

- ☐ Abdomen
- ☐ Joints
- ☐ Stomach
- ☐ Rectum
- ☐ Other ______

Notes

Other Symptoms

- ☐ Bloating
- ☐ Fatigue
- ☐ Nausea
- ☐ Flatulence
- ☐ Vomiting
- ☐ Other ______

Stress Level

Sleep

Energy Level

Activity Level

Medications

______

______

______

______

______

Daily Tracking

DATE:

S M T W T F S

Fluid Tracker 8 oz 8 oz 8 oz 8 oz 8 oz 8 oz 8 oz 8 oz

Meal Tracking

Time	Meal	Pain Scale 0-5 0= No pain 5= Severe
BREAKFAST		
LUNCH		
DINNER		
SNACKS		

Bowel Activity

Normal	Very Hard	Abnormalities
		Blood Mucus Other
		Blood Mucus Other
		Blood Mucus Other
		Blood Mucus Other
	More?	

Other Symptoms

- ☐ Bloating
- ☐ Fatigue
- ☐ Nausea
- ☐ Flatulence
- ☐ Vomiting
- ☐ Other ______

Stress Level

Sleep

Energy Level

Activity Level

Pain Location (If Applicable)

- ☐ Abdomen
- ☐ Joints
- ☐ Stomach
- ☐ Rectum
- ☐ Other ______

Medications

Notes

Daily Tracking

DATE:

S M T W T F S

Fluid Tracker 8 oz 8 oz 8 oz 8 oz 8 oz 8 oz 8 oz 8 oz

Meal Tracking

Time	Meal	Pain Scale 0-5 0= No pain 5= Severe
BREAKFAST		
LUNCH		
DINNER		
SNACKS		

Bowel Activity

Normal	Very Hard	Abnormalities
		☐ Blood ☐ Mucus ☐ Other ______
		☐ Blood ☐ Mucus ☐ Other ______
		☐ Blood ☐ Mucus ☐ Other ______
		☐ Blood ☐ Mucus ☐ Other ______
	More?	

Other Symptoms

☐ Bloating ☐ Fatigue
☐ Nausea ☐ Flatulence
☐ Vomiting
☐ Other ______________________

Stress Level

Sleep

Energy Level

Activity Level

Pain Location (If Applicable)

☐ Abdomen ☐ Joints
☐ Stomach ☐ Rectum
☐ Other ______________________

Medications

____
____
____
____
____

Notes

Daily Tracking

DATE:

S M T W T F S

Fluid Tracker 8 oz | 8 oz | 8 oz | 8 oz | 8 oz | 8 oz | 8 oz | 8 oz

Meal Tracking

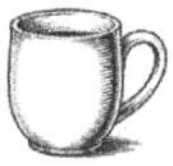

Time	Meal	Pain Scale 0-5 0= No pain 5= Severe
BREAKFAST		
LUNCH		
DINNER		
SNACKS		

Bowel Activity

Normal	Very Hard	Abnormalities
		☐ Blood ☐ Mucus ☐ Other ______
		☐ Blood ☐ Mucus ☐ Other ______
		☐ Blood ☐ Mucus ☐ Other ______
		☐ Blood ☐ Mucus ☐ Other ______
	More?	

Other Symptoms

☐ Bloating ☐ Fatigue
☐ Nausea ☐ Flatulence
☐ Vomiting
☐ Other ______________________

Stress Level

Sleep

Energy Level

Activity Level

Pain Location (If Applicable)

☐ Abdomen ☐ Joints
☐ Stomach ☐ Rectum
☐ Other ______________________

Medications

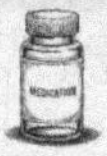

____
____
____
____
____

Notes

Daily Tracking

DATE:

S M T W T F S

Fluid Tracker: 8 oz | 8 oz | 8 oz | 8 oz | 8 oz | 8 oz | 8 oz | 8 oz

Meal Tracking

Time	Meal	Pain Scale 0-5 0= No pain 5= Severe
BREAKFAST		
LUNCH		
DINNER		
SNACKS		

Bowel Activity

Normal	Very Hard	Abnormalities
		☐ Blood ☐ Mucus ☐ Other ______
		☐ Blood ☐ Mucus ☐ Other ______
		☐ Blood ☐ Mucus ☐ Other ______
		☐ Blood ☐ Mucus ☐ Other ______
	More?	

Other Symptoms

- ☐ Bloating
- ☐ Fatigue
- ☐ Nausea
- ☐ Flatulence
- ☐ Vomiting
- ☐ Other ______________________

Stress Level

Sleep

Energy Level

Activity Level

Pain Location (If Applicable)

- ☐ Abdomen
- ☐ Joints
- ☐ Stomach
- ☐ Rectum
- ☐ Other ______________________

Notes

Medications

____

____

____

____

____

Daily Tracking

DATE:

S M T W T F S

Fluid Tracker: 8 oz | 8 oz | 8 oz | 8 oz | 8 oz | 8 oz | 8 oz | 8 oz

Meal Tracking

Time	Meal	Pain Scale 0-5 0= No pain 5= Severe
BREAKFAST		
LUNCH		
DINNER		
SNACKS		

Bowel Activity

Normal	Very Hard	Abnormalities
		☐ Blood ☐ Mucus ☐ Other ______
		☐ Blood ☐ Mucus ☐ Other ______
		☐ Blood ☐ Mucus ☐ Other ______
		☐ Blood ☐ Mucus ☐ Other ______
	More?	

Other Symptoms

- ☐ Bloating
- ☐ Fatigue
- ☐ Nausea
- ☐ Flatulence
- ☐ Vomiting
- ☐ Other ______________________

Stress Level

Sleep

Energy Level

Activity Level

Pain Location (If Applicable)

- ☐ Abdomen
- ☐ Joints
- ☐ Stomach
- ☐ Rectum
- ☐ Other ______________________

Medications

____

____

____

____

____

Notes

Weekly Reflections

What was the best thing that happened this week?

What was the hardest thing that happened this week?

What helped you the most this week?

What gave you hope this week?

What's one small win you can celebrate?

Was there something that eased your stress?

Overall, this week I felt

☐ A little better ☐ A lot better ☐ A little worse ☐ A lot worse

☐ About the same

Next week I want to:

____

____

____

____

Remember, strength isn't about pushing harder. Sometimes, it's about giving yourself grace.

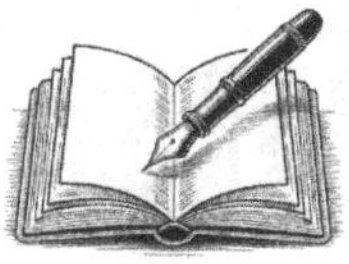

Daily Tracking

DATE:

S M T W T F S

Fluid Tracker: 8 oz | 8 oz | 8 oz | 8 oz | 8 oz | 8 oz | 8 oz | 8 oz

Meal Tracking

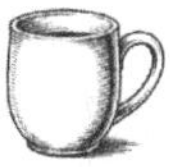

Time	Meal	Pain Scale 0-5 0= No pain 5= Severe
BREAKFAST		
LUNCH		
DINNER		
SNACKS		

Bowel Activity

Normal	Very Hard	Abnormalities
		☐ Blood ☐ Mucus ☐ Other ______
		☐ Blood ☐ Mucus ☐ Other ______
		☐ Blood ☐ Mucus ☐ Other ______
		☐ Blood ☐ Mucus ☐ Other ______
	More?	

Other Symptoms

- ☐ Bloating
- ☐ Fatigue
- ☐ Nausea
- ☐ Flatulence
- ☐ Vomiting
- ☐ Other ______________________

Stress Level

Sleep

Energy Level

Activity Level

Pain Location (If Applicable)

- ☐ Abdomen
- ☐ Joints
- ☐ Stomach
- ☐ Rectum
- ☐ Other ______________________

Medications

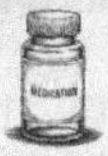

____

____

____

____

____

Notes

Daily Tracking

DATE:

S M T W T F S

Fluid Tracker: 8 oz | 8 oz | 8 oz | 8 oz | 8 oz | 8 oz | 8 oz | 8 oz

Meal Tracking

Time	Meal	Pain Scale 0-5 0= No pain 5= Severe
BREAKFAST		
LUNCH		
DINNER		
SNACKS		

Bowel Activity

Normal	Very Hard	Abnormalities
		☐ Blood ☐ Mucus ☐ Other ______
		☐ Blood ☐ Mucus ☐ Other ______
		☐ Blood ☐ Mucus ☐ Other ______
		☐ Blood ☐ Mucus ☐ Other ______
	More?	

Other Symptoms

☐ Bloating
☐ Fatigue
☐ Nausea
☐ Flatulence
☐ Vomiting
☐ Other ______________________

Stress Level

Sleep

Energy Level

Activity Level

Pain Location (If Applicable)

☐ Abdomen
☐ Joints
☐ Stomach
☐ Rectum
☐ Other ______________________

Medications

____
____
____
____
____

Notes

Daily Tracking

DATE:

S M T W T F S

Meal Tracking

Fluid Tracker: 8 oz | 8 oz | 8 oz | 8 oz | 8 oz | 8 oz | 8 oz | 8 oz

Time	Meal	Pain Scale 0-5 0= No pain 5= Severe
BREAKFAST		
LUNCH		
DINNER		
SNACKS		

Bowel Activity

Normal	Very Hard	Abnormalities
		☐ Blood ☐ Mucus ☐ Other ______
		☐ Blood ☐ Mucus ☐ Other ______
		☐ Blood ☐ Mucus ☐ Other ______
		☐ Blood ☐ Mucus ☐ Other ______
	More?	

Other Symptoms

- ☐ Bloating
- ☐ Fatigue
- ☐ Nausea
- ☐ Flatulence
- ☐ Vomiting
- ☐ Other ______________________

Stress Level

Sleep

Energy Level

Activity Level

Pain Location (If Applicable)

- ☐ Abdomen
- ☐ Joints
- ☐ Stomach
- ☐ Rectum
- ☐ Other ______________________

Medications

____

____

____

____

____

Notes

Daily Tracking

DATE:

S M T W T F S

Fluid Tracker 8 oz 8 oz 8 oz 8 oz 8 oz 8 oz 8 oz 8 oz

Meal Tracking

Time	Meal	Pain Scale 0-5 0= No pain 5= Severe
BREAKFAST		
LUNCH		
DINNER		
SNACKS		

Bowel Activity

Normal	Very Hard	Abnormalities
		☐ Blood ☐ Mucus ☐ Other ____
		☐ Blood ☐ Mucus ☐ Other ____
		☐ Blood ☐ Mucus ☐ Other ____
		☐ Blood ☐ Mucus ☐ Other ____
	More?	

Other Symptoms

- ☐ Bloating
- ☐ Fatigue
- ☐ Nausea
- ☐ Flatulence
- ☐ Vomiting
- ☐ Other ____________________

Stress Level

Sleep

Energy Level

Activity Level

Pain Location (If Applicable)

- ☐ Abdomen
- ☐ Joints
- ☐ Stomach
- ☐ Rectum
- ☐ Other ____________________

Medications

Notes

Daily Tracking

DATE:

S M T W T F S

Fluid Tracker 8 oz | 8 oz | 8 oz | 8 oz | 8 oz | 8 oz | 8 oz | 8 oz

Meal Tracking

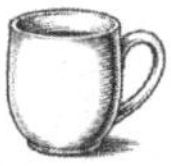

Time	Meal	Pain Scale 0-5 0= No pain 5= Severe
BREAKFAST		
LUNCH		
DINNER		
SNACKS		

Bowel Activity

Normal	Very Hard	Abnormalities
		☐ Blood ☐ Mucus ☐ Other ______
		☐ Blood ☐ Mucus ☐ Other ______
		☐ Blood ☐ Mucus ☐ Other ______
		☐ Blood ☐ Mucus ☐ Other ______
	More?	

Other Symptoms

- ☐ Bloating
- ☐ Fatigue
- ☐ Nausea
- ☐ Flatulence
- ☐ Vomiting
- ☐ Other ______

Stress Level

Sleep

Energy Level

Activity Level

Pain Location (If Applicable)

- ☐ Abdomen
- ☐ Joints
- ☐ Stomach
- ☐ Rectum
- ☐ Other ______

Notes

Medications

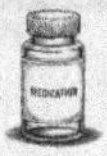

______

______

______

______

______

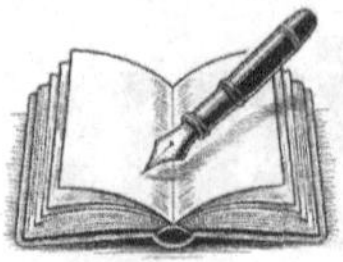

Daily Tracking

DATE:	S M T W T F S

Fluid Tracker 8 oz 8 oz 8 oz 8 oz 8 oz 8 oz 8 oz 8 oz

Meal Tracking

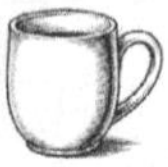

Time	Meal	Pain Scale 0-5 0= No pain 5= Severe
BREAKFAST		
LUNCH		
DINNER		
SNACKS		

Bowel Activity

Normal	Very Hard	Abnormalities
		☐ Blood ☐ Mucus ☐ Other ______
		☐ Blood ☐ Mucus ☐ Other ______
		☐ Blood ☐ Mucus ☐ Other ______
		☐ Blood ☐ Mucus ☐ Other ______
	More?	

Other Symptoms

☐ Bloating ☐ Fatigue
☐ Nausea ☐ Flatulence
☐ Vomiting
☐ Other ______________________

Stress Level

Sleep

Energy Level

Activity Level

Pain Location (If Applicable)

☐ Abdomen ☐ Joints
☐ Stomach ☐ Rectum
☐ Other ______________________

Notes

Medications

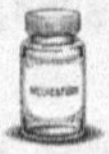

____
____
____
____
____

Daily Tracking

DATE:

S M T W T F S

Fluid Tracker: 8 oz | 8 oz | 8 oz | 8 oz | 8 oz | 8 oz | 8 oz | 8 oz

Meal Tracking

Time	Meal	Pain Scale 0-5 0= No pain 5= Severe
BREAKFAST		
LUNCH		
DINNER		
SNACKS		

Bowel Activity

Normal	Very Hard	Abnormalities
		☐ Blood ☐ Mucus ☐ Other ______
		☐ Blood ☐ Mucus ☐ Other ______
		☐ Blood ☐ Mucus ☐ Other ______
		☐ Blood ☐ Mucus ☐ Other ______
	More?	

Other Symptoms

- ☐ Bloating
- ☐ Fatigue
- ☐ Nausea
- ☐ Flatulence
- ☐ Vomiting
- ☐ Other ______________________

Stress Level

Sleep

Energy Level

Activity Level

Pain Location (If Applicable)

- ☐ Abdomen
- ☐ Joints
- ☐ Stomach
- ☐ Rectum
- ☐ Other ______________________

Medications

____

____

____

____

____

Notes

Weekly Reflections

What was the best thing that happened this week?

What was the hardest thing that happened this week?

What helped you the most this week?

What gave you hope this week?

What's one small win you can celebrate?

Was there something that eased your stress?

Overall, this week I felt

☐ A little better ☐ A lot better ☐ A little worse ☐ A lot worse
☐ About the same

Next week I want to:

____

____

____

____

Remember, strength isn't about pushing harder.
Sometimes, it's about giving yourself grace.

Daily Tracking

DATE:

S M T W T F S

Meal Tracking

Fluid Tracker: 8 oz | 8 oz | 8 oz | 8 oz | 8 oz | 8 oz | 8 oz | 8 oz

Time	Meal	Pain Scale 0-5 0= No pain 5= Severe
BREAKFAST		
LUNCH		
DINNER		
SNACKS		

Bowel Activity

Normal	Very Hard	Abnormalities
		☐ Blood ☐ Mucus ☐ Other ______
		☐ Blood ☐ Mucus ☐ Other ______
		☐ Blood ☐ Mucus ☐ Other ______
		☐ Blood ☐ Mucus ☐ Other ______
	More?	

Other Symptoms

- ☐ Bloating
- ☐ Fatigue
- ☐ Nausea
- ☐ Flatulence
- ☐ Vomiting
- ☐ Other ______________________

Stress Level

Sleep

Energy Level

Activity Level

Pain Location (If Applicable)

- ☐ Abdomen
- ☐ Joints
- ☐ Stomach
- ☐ Rectum
- ☐ Other ______________________

Notes

Medications

____

____

____

____

____

Daily Tracking

DATE:

S M T W T F S

Fluid Tracker 8 oz 8 oz 8 oz 8 oz 8 oz 8 oz 8 oz 8 oz

Meal Tracking

Time	Meal	Pain Scale 0-5 0= No pain 5= Severe
BREAKFAST		
LUNCH		
DINNER		
SNACKS		

Bowel Activity

Normal	Very Hard	Abnormalities
		☐ Blood ☐ Mucus ☐ Other ______
		☐ Blood ☐ Mucus ☐ Other ______
		☐ Blood ☐ Mucus ☐ Other ______
		☐ Blood ☐ Mucus ☐ Other ______
	More?	

Other Symptoms

- ☐ Bloating
- ☐ Fatigue
- ☐ Nausea
- ☐ Flatulence
- ☐ Vomiting
- ☐ Other ______

Stress Level

Sleep

Energy Level

Activity Level

Pain Location (If Applicable)

- ☐ Abdomen
- ☐ Joints
- ☐ Stomach
- ☐ Rectum
- ☐ Other ______

Medications

______
______
______
______
______

Notes

Daily Tracking

DATE:

S M T W T F S

Meal Tracking

Fluid Tracker: 8 oz 8 oz 8 oz 8 oz 8 oz 8 oz 8 oz 8 oz

Time	Meal	Pain Scale 0-5 0= No pain 5= Severe
BREAKFAST		
LUNCH		
DINNER		
SNACKS		

Bowel Activity

Normal	Very Hard	Abnormalities
		☐ Blood ☐ Mucus ☐ Other ______
		☐ Blood ☐ Mucus ☐ Other ______
		☐ Blood ☐ Mucus ☐ Other ______
		☐ Blood ☐ Mucus ☐ Other ______
	More?	

Other Symptoms

☐ Bloating ☐ Fatigue
☐ Nausea ☐ Flatulence
☐ Vomiting
☐ Other ______

Stress Level

Sleep

Energy Level

Activity Level

Pain Location (If Applicable)

☐ Abdomen ☐ Joints
☐ Stomach ☐ Rectum
☐ Other ______

Medications

Notes

Daily Tracking

DATE:

S M T W T F S

Meal Tracking

Fluid Tracker: 8 oz | 8 oz | 8 oz | 8 oz | 8 oz | 8 oz | 8 oz | 8 oz

Time	Meal	Pain Scale 0-5 0= No pain 5= Severe
BREAKFAST		
LUNCH		
DINNER		
SNACKS		

Bowel Activity

Normal	Very Hard	Abnormalities
		☐ Blood ☐ Mucus ☐ Other ______
		☐ Blood ☐ Mucus ☐ Other ______
		☐ Blood ☐ Mucus ☐ Other ______
		☐ Blood ☐ Mucus ☐ Other ______
	More?	

Other Symptoms

☐ Bloating ☐ Fatigue
☐ Nausea ☐ Flatulence
☐ Vomiting
☐ Other ______

Stress Level

Sleep

Energy Level

Activity Level

Pain Location (If Applicable)

☐ Abdomen ☐ Joints
☐ Stomach ☐ Rectum
☐ Other ______

Medications

Notes

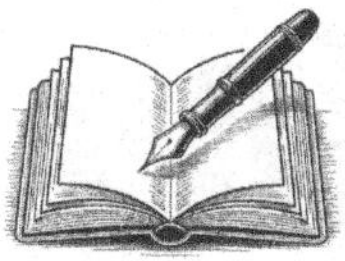

Daily Tracking

DATE:

S M T W T F S

Meal Tracking

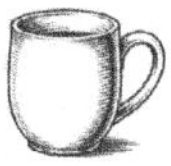

Fluid Tracker 8 oz 8 oz 8 oz 8 oz 8 oz 8 oz 8 oz 8 oz

Time	Meal	Pain Scale 0-5 0= No pain 5= Severe
BREAKFAST		
LUNCH		
DINNER		
SNACKS		

Bowel Activity

Normal	Very Hard	Abnormalities
		☐ Blood ☐ Mucus ☐ Other ______
		☐ Blood ☐ Mucus ☐ Other ______
		☐ Blood ☐ Mucus ☐ Other ______
		☐ Blood ☐ Mucus ☐ Other ______
	More?	

Other Symptoms

☐ Bloating ☐ Fatigue
☐ Nausea ☐ Flatulence
☐ Vomiting
☐ Other ______________________

Stress Level

Sleep

Energy Level

Activity Level

Pain Location (If Applicable)

☐ Abdomen ☐ Joints
☐ Stomach ☐ Rectum
☐ Other ______________________

Medications

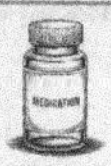

____
____
____
____
____

Notes

Daily Tracking

DATE:

S M T W T F S

Fluid Tracker: 8 oz | 8 oz | 8 oz | 8 oz | 8 oz | 8 oz | 8 oz | 8 oz

Meal Tracking

Time	Meal	Pain Scale 0-5 0= No pain 5= Severe
BREAKFAST		
LUNCH		
DINNER		
SNACKS		

Bowel Activity

Normal	Very Hard	Abnormalities
		☐ Blood ☐ Mucus ☐ Other ______
		☐ Blood ☐ Mucus ☐ Other ______
		☐ Blood ☐ Mucus ☐ Other ______
		☐ Blood ☐ Mucus ☐ Other ______
	More?	

Other Symptoms

☐ Bloating ☐ Fatigue
☐ Nausea ☐ Flatulence
☐ Vomiting
☐ Other ______________________

Stress Level

Sleep

Energy Level

Activity Level

Pain Location (If Applicable)

☐ Abdomen ☐ Joints
☐ Stomach ☐ Rectum
☐ Other ______________________

Medications

____
____
____
____
____

Notes

Daily Tracking

DATE:

S M T W T F S

Fluid Tracker: 8 oz | 8 oz | 8 oz | 8 oz | 8 oz | 8 oz | 8 oz | 8 oz

Meal Tracking

Time	Meal	Pain Scale 0-5 0= No pain 5= Severe
BREAKFAST		
LUNCH		
DINNER		
SNACKS		

Bowel Activity

Normal	Very Hard	Abnormalities
		☐ Blood ☐ Mucus ☐ Other ____
		☐ Blood ☐ Mucus ☐ Other ____
		☐ Blood ☐ Mucus ☐ Other ____
		☐ Blood ☐ Mucus ☐ Other ____
	More?	

Other Symptoms

- ☐ Bloating
- ☐ Fatigue
- ☐ Nausea
- ☐ Flatulence
- ☐ Vomiting
- ☐ Other ____

Stress Level

Sleep

Energy Level

Activity Level

Pain Location (If Applicable)

- ☐ Abdomen
- ☐ Joints
- ☐ Stomach
- ☐ Rectum
- ☐ Other ____

Medications

Notes

Weekly Reflections

What was the best thing that happened this week?

What was the hardest thing that happened this week?

What helped you the most this week?

What gave you hope this week?

What's one small win you can celebrate?

Was there something that eased your stress?

Overall, this week I felt

☐ A little better ☐ A lot better ☐ A little worse ☐ A lot worse

☐ About the same

Next week I want to:

____

____

____

____

IMPORTANT REMINDER

You are more than symptoms. Celebrate what brings you joy, however small.

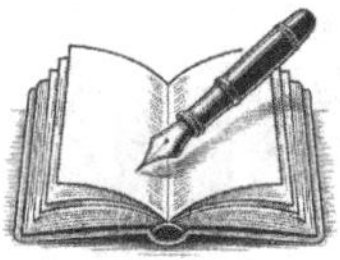

Daily Tracking

DATE:

S M T W T F S

Fluid Tracker 8 oz 8 oz 8 oz 8 oz 8 oz 8 oz 8 oz 8 oz

Meal Tracking

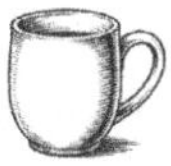

Time	Meal	Pain Scale 0-5 0= No pain 5= Severe
BREAKFAST		
LUNCH		
DINNER		
SNACKS		

Bowel Activity

Normal	Very Hard	Abnormalities
		☐ Blood ☐ Mucus ☐ Other ______
		☐ Blood ☐ Mucus ☐ Other ______
		☐ Blood ☐ Mucus ☐ Other ______
		☐ Blood ☐ Mucus ☐ Other ______
	More?	

Other Symptoms

☐ Bloating ☐ Fatigue
☐ Nausea ☐ Flatulence
☐ Vomiting
☐ Other ______________________

Stress Level

Sleep

Energy Level

Activity Level

Pain Location (If Applicable)

☐ Abdomen ☐ Joints
☐ Stomach ☐ Rectum
☐ Other ______________________

Medications

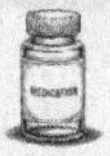

____
____
____
____
____

Notes

Daily Tracking

DATE:

S M T W T F S

Fluid Tracker: 8 oz | 8 oz | 8 oz | 8 oz | 8 oz | 8 oz | 8 oz | 8 oz

Meal Tracking

Time	Meal	Pain Scale 0-5 0= No pain 5= Severe
BREAKFAST		
LUNCH		
DINNER		
SNACKS		

Bowel Activity

Normal	Very Hard	Abnormalities
		☐ Blood ☐ Mucus ☐ Other ______
		☐ Blood ☐ Mucus ☐ Other ______
		☐ Blood ☐ Mucus ☐ Other ______
		☐ Blood ☐ Mucus ☐ Other ______
	More?	

Other Symptoms

☐ Bloating ☐ Fatigue
☐ Nausea ☐ Flatulence
☐ Vomiting
☐ Other ______________________

Stress Level

Sleep

Energy Level

Activity Level

Pain Location (If Applicable)

☐ Abdomen ☐ Joints
☐ Stomach ☐ Rectum
☐ Other ______________________

Medications

____
____
____
____
____

Notes

Daily Tracking

DATE:

S M T W T F S

Fluid Tracker: 8 oz 8 oz 8 oz 8 oz 8 oz 8 oz 8 oz 8 oz

Meal Tracking

Time	Meal	Pain Scale 0-5 0= No pain 5= Severe
BREAKFAST		
LUNCH		
DINNER		
SNACKS		

Bowel Activity

Normal	Very Hard	Abnormalities
		☐ Blood ☐ Mucus ☐ Other ____
		☐ Blood ☐ Mucus ☐ Other ____
		☐ Blood ☐ Mucus ☐ Other ____
		☐ Blood ☐ Mucus ☐ Other ____
	More?	

Other Symptoms

- ☐ Bloating
- ☐ Fatigue
- ☐ Nausea
- ☐ Flatulence
- ☐ Vomiting
- ☐ Other ______________________

Stress Level

Sleep

Energy Level

Activity Level

Pain Location (If Applicable)

- ☐ Abdomen
- ☐ Joints
- ☐ Stomach
- ☐ Rectum
- ☐ Other ______________________

Medications

____

____

____

____

____

Notes

Daily Tracking

DATE:

S M T W T F S

Fluid Tracker 8 oz 8 oz 8 oz 8 oz 8 oz 8 oz 8 oz 8 oz

Meal Tracking

Time	Meal	Pain Scale 0-5 0= No pain 5= Severe
BREAKFAST		
LUNCH		
DINNER		
SNACKS		

Bowel Activity

Normal	Very Hard	Abnormalities
		☐ Blood ☐ Mucus ☐ Other ____
		☐ Blood ☐ Mucus ☐ Other ____
		☐ Blood ☐ Mucus ☐ Other ____
		☐ Blood ☐ Mucus ☐ Other ____
	More?	

Other Symptoms

☐ Bloating ☐ Fatigue
☐ Nausea ☐ Flatulence
☐ Vomiting
☐ Other ____________________

Stress Level

Sleep

Energy Level

Activity Level

Pain Location (If Applicable)

☐ Abdomen ☐ Joints
☐ Stomach ☐ Rectum
☐ Other ____________________

Medications

____
____
____
____
____

Notes

Daily Tracking

DATE:

S M T W T F S

Fluid Tracker: 8 oz | 8 oz | 8 oz | 8 oz | 8 oz | 8 oz | 8 oz | 8 oz

Meal Tracking

Time	Meal	Pain Scale 0-5 0= No pain 5= Severe
BREAKFAST		
LUNCH		
DINNER		
SNACKS		

Bowel Activity

Normal	Very Hard	Abnormalities
		☐ Blood ☐ Mucus ☐ Other ______
		☐ Blood ☐ Mucus ☐ Other ______
		☐ Blood ☐ Mucus ☐ Other ______
		☐ Blood ☐ Mucus ☐ Other ______
	More?	

Other Symptoms

- ☐ Bloating
- ☐ Fatigue
- ☐ Nausea
- ☐ Flatulence
- ☐ Vomiting
- ☐ Other ______

Stress Level

Sleep

Energy Level

Activity Level

Pain Location (If Applicable)

- ☐ Abdomen
- ☐ Joints
- ☐ Stomach
- ☐ Rectum
- ☐ Other ______

Medications

______

______

______

______

______

Notes

Daily Tracking

DATE:

S M T W T F S

Fluid Tracker 8 oz 8 oz 8 oz 8 oz 8 oz 8 oz 8 oz 8 oz

Meal Tracking

Time	Meal	Pain Scale 0-5 0= No pain 5= Severe
BREAKFAST		
LUNCH		
DINNER		
SNACKS		

Bowel Activity

Normal	Very Hard	Abnormalities
		☐ Blood ☐ Mucus ☐ Other
		☐ Blood ☐ Mucus ☐ Other
		☐ Blood ☐ Mucus ☐ Other
		☐ Blood ☐ Mucus ☐ Other
	More?	

Other Symptoms

☐ Bloating ☐ Fatigue
☐ Nausea ☐ Flatulence
☐ Vomiting
☐ Other ____________

Stress Level

Sleep

Energy Level

Activity Level

Pain Location (If Applicable)

☐ Abdomen ☐ Joints
☐ Stomach ☐ Rectum
☐ Other ____________

Medications

Notes

Daily Tracking

DATE:

S M T W T F S

Fluid Tracker: 8 oz | 8 oz | 8 oz | 8 oz | 8 oz | 8 oz | 8 oz | 8 oz

Meal Tracking

Time	Meal	Pain Scale 0-5 0= No pain 5= Severe
BREAKFAST		
LUNCH		
DINNER		
SNACKS		

Bowel Activity

Normal	Very Hard	Abnormalities
		☐ Blood ☐ Mucus ☐ Other ______
		☐ Blood ☐ Mucus ☐ Other ______
		☐ Blood ☐ Mucus ☐ Other ______
		☐ Blood ☐ Mucus ☐ Other ______
	More?	

Other Symptoms

- ☐ Bloating
- ☐ Fatigue
- ☐ Nausea
- ☐ Flatulence
- ☐ Vomiting
- ☐ Other ______________________

Stress Level

Sleep

Energy Level

Activity Level

Pain Location (If Applicable)

- ☐ Abdomen
- ☐ Joints
- ☐ Stomach
- ☐ Rectum
- ☐ Other ______________________

Medications

Notes

Weekly Reflections

What was the best thing that happened this week?

What was the hardest thing that happened this week?

What helped you the most this week?

What gave you hope this week?

What's one small win you can celebrate?

Was there something that eased your stress?

Overall, this week I felt

☐ A little better ☐ A lot better ☐ A little worse ☐ A lot worse

☐ About the same

Next week I want to:

____

____

____

____

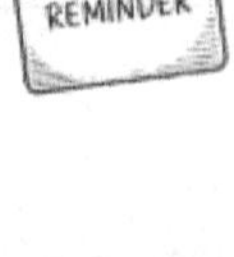

The fact that you are here, reflecting, shows resilience. That's something to be proud of.

Monthly Thoughts

This page is your space to step back and see the bigger picture. Each month brings its own challenges and small victories—use this space to notice patterns, celebrate progress, and reflect on what your body and mind are teaching you. These notes can guide you forward with greater clarity and self-compassion.

This Month I Noticed...

(Write down patterns in your symptoms, energy, or mood.)

Biggest Challenge: ______________________________

____

Brightest Moment: ______________________________

____

Triggers I Noticed: ______________________________

____

Things That Helped: ______________________________

____

Medication / Treatment Notes: (Any changes, side effects, or adjustments.) ______________________________

____

____

Self-Care Check-In

How well I cared for myself this month: ______________________________

____

Looking Forward

Next month I want to focus on: ______________________________

____

____

Symptom Overview

Good Days: ________ Mild Days: ________ Flare Days: ________

IMPORTANT REMINDER

Healing is stitched together one small choice at a time.

Daily Tracking

DATE:

S M T W T F S

Fluid Tracker: 8 oz | 8 oz | 8 oz | 8 oz | 8 oz | 8 oz | 8 oz | 8 oz

Meal Tracking

Time	Meal	Pain Scale 0-5 0= No pain 5= Severe
BREAKFAST		
LUNCH		
DINNER		
SNACKS		

Bowel Activity

Normal	Very Hard	Abnormalities
		☐ Blood ☐ Mucus ☐ Other ____
		☐ Blood ☐ Mucus ☐ Other ____
		☐ Blood ☐ Mucus ☐ Other ____
		☐ Blood ☐ Mucus ☐ Other ____
	More?	

Other Symptoms

☐ Bloating ☐ Fatigue
☐ Nausea ☐ Flatulence
☐ Vomiting
☐ Other ____

Stress Level

Sleep

Energy Level

Activity Level

Pain Location (If Applicable)

☐ Abdomen ☐ Joints
☐ Stomach ☐ Rectum
☐ Other ____

Medications

Notes

Daily Tracking

DATE:

S M T W T F S

Fluid Tracker: 8 oz | 8 oz | 8 oz | 8 oz | 8 oz | 8 oz | 8 oz | 8 oz

Meal Tracking

Time	Meal	Pain Scale 0-5 0= No pain 5= Severe
BREAKFAST		
LUNCH		
DINNER		
SNACKS		

Bowel Activity

Normal	Very Hard	Abnormalities
		☐ Blood ☐ Mucus ☐ Other ____
		☐ Blood ☐ Mucus ☐ Other ____
		☐ Blood ☐ Mucus ☐ Other ____
		☐ Blood ☐ Mucus ☐ Other ____
	More?	

Other Symptoms

☐ Bloating ☐ Fatigue
☐ Nausea ☐ Flatulence
☐ Vomiting
☐ Other ____________________

Stress Level

Sleep

Energy Level

Activity Level

Pain Location (If Applicable)

☐ Abdomen ☐ Joints
☐ Stomach ☐ Rectum
☐ Other ____________________

Medications

____
____
____
____
____

Notes

Daily Tracking

DATE:

S M T W T F S

Meal Tracking

Fluid Tracker: 8 oz | 8 oz | 8 oz | 8 oz | 8 oz | 8 oz | 8 oz | 8 oz

Time	Meal	Pain Scale 0-5 0= No pain 5= Severe
BREAKFAST		
LUNCH		
DINNER		
SNACKS		

Bowel Activity

Normal	Very Hard	Abnormalities
		☐ Blood ☐ Mucus ☐ Other ______
		☐ Blood ☐ Mucus ☐ Other ______
		☐ Blood ☐ Mucus ☐ Other ______
		☐ Blood ☐ Mucus ☐ Other ______
	More?	

Pain Location (If Applicable)

- ☐ Abdomen
- ☐ Joints
- ☐ Stomach
- ☐ Rectum
- ☐ Other ______________________

Notes

Other Symptoms

- ☐ Bloating
- ☐ Fatigue
- ☐ Nausea
- ☐ Flatulence
- ☐ Vomiting
- ☐ Other ______________________

Stress Level

Sleep

Energy Level

Activity Level

Medications

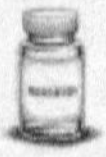

____

____

____

____

____

Daily Tracking

DATE:

S M T W T F S

Fluid Tracker: 8 oz | 8 oz | 8 oz | 8 oz | 8 oz | 8 oz | 8 oz | 8 oz

Meal Tracking

Time	Meal	Pain Scale 0-5 0= No pain 5= Severe
BREAKFAST		
LUNCH		
DINNER		
SNACKS		

Bowel Activity

Normal	Very Hard	Abnormalities
		☐ Blood ☐ Mucus ☐ Other ______
		☐ Blood ☐ Mucus ☐ Other ______
		☐ Blood ☐ Mucus ☐ Other ______
		☐ Blood ☐ Mucus ☐ Other ______
	More?	

Other Symptoms

☐ Bloating ☐ Fatigue
☐ Nausea ☐ Flatulence
☐ Vomiting
☐ Other ______________________

Stress Level

Sleep

Energy Level

Activity Level

Pain Location (If Applicable)

☐ Abdomen ☐ Joints
☐ Stomach ☐ Rectum
☐ Other ______________________

Medications

____
____
____
____
____

Notes

Daily Tracking

DATE:

S M T W T F S

Fluid Tracker: 8 oz 8 oz 8 oz 8 oz 8 oz 8 oz 8 oz 8 oz

Meal Tracking

Time	Meal	Pain Scale 0-5 0= No pain 5= Severe
BREAKFAST		
LUNCH		
DINNER		
SNACKS		

Bowel Activity

Normal	Very Hard	Abnormalities
		☐ Blood ☐ Mucus ☐ Other ______
		☐ Blood ☐ Mucus ☐ Other ______
		☐ Blood ☐ Mucus ☐ Other ______
		☐ Blood ☐ Mucus ☐ Other ______
	More?	

Other Symptoms

☐ Bloating ☐ Fatigue
☐ Nausea ☐ Flatulence
☐ Vomiting
☐ Other ______________________

Stress Level

Sleep

Energy Level

Activity Level

Pain Location (If Applicable)

☐ Abdomen ☐ Joints
☐ Stomach ☐ Rectum
☐ Other ______________________

Notes

Medications

____

____

____

____

____

Daily Tracking

DATE:

S M T W T F S

Fluid Tracker: 8 oz | 8 oz | 8 oz | 8 oz | 8 oz | 8 oz | 8 oz | 8 oz

Meal Tracking

Time	Meal	Pain Scale 0-5 0= No pain 5= Severe
BREAKFAST		
LUNCH		
DINNER		
SNACKS		

Bowel Activity

Normal → Very Hard		Abnormalities
		☐ Blood ☐ Mucus ☐ Other ______
		☐ Blood ☐ Mucus ☐ Other ______
		☐ Blood ☐ Mucus ☐ Other ______
		☐ Blood ☐ Mucus ☐ Other ______
	More?	

Other Symptoms

☐ Bloating ☐ Fatigue
☐ Nausea ☐ Flatulence
☐ Vomiting
☐ Other ______________________

Stress Level

Sleep

Energy Level

Activity Level

Pain Location (If Applicable)

☐ Abdomen ☐ Joints
☐ Stomach ☐ Rectum
☐ Other ______________________

Medications

____
____
____
____
____

Notes

Daily Tracking

DATE:

S M T W T F S

Fluid Tracker 8 oz 8 oz 8 oz 8 oz 8 oz 8 oz 8 oz 8 oz

Meal Tracking

Time	Meal	Pain Scale 0-5 0= No pain 5= Severe
BREAKFAST		
LUNCH		
DINNER		
SNACKS		

Bowel Activity

Normal	Very Hard	Abnormalities
		☐ Blood ☐ Mucus ☐ Other ______
		☐ Blood ☐ Mucus ☐ Other ______
		☐ Blood ☐ Mucus ☐ Other ______
		☐ Blood ☐ Mucus ☐ Other ______
	More?	

Other Symptoms

☐ Bloating ☐ Fatigue
☐ Nausea ☐ Flatulence
☐ Vomiting
☐ Other ______

Stress Level

Sleep

Energy Level

Activity Leve

Pain Location (If Applicable)

☐ Abdomen ☐ Joints
☐ Stomach ☐ Rectum
☐ Other ______

Medications

Notes

Weekly Reflections

What was the best thing that happened this week?

What was the hardest thing that happened this week?

What helped you the most this week?

What gave you hope this week?

What's one small win you can celebrate?

Was there something that eased your stress?

Overall, this week I felt

☐ A little better ☐ A lot better ☐ A little worse ☐ A lot worse

☐ About the same

Next week I want to:

____

____

____

____

This week may carry challenges, but it also holds space for kindness toward yourself.

Daily Tracking

DATE:

S M T W T F S

Fluid Tracker 8 oz 8 oz 8 oz 8 oz 8 oz 8 oz 8 oz 8 oz

Meal Tracking

Time	Meal	Pain Scale 0-5 0= No pain 5= Severe
BREAKFAST		
LUNCH		
DINNER		
SNACKS		

Bowel Activity

Normal	Very Hard	Abnormalities
		☐ Blood ☐ Mucus ☐ Other ______
		☐ Blood ☐ Mucus ☐ Other ______
		☐ Blood ☐ Mucus ☐ Other ______
		☐ Blood ☐ Mucus ☐ Other ______
	More?	

Other Symptoms

☐ Bloating ☐ Fatigue
☐ Nausea ☐ Flatulence
☐ Vomiting
☐ Other ______________________

Stress Level

Sleep

Energy Level

Activity Level

Pain Location (If Applicable)

☐ Abdomen ☐ Joints
☐ Stomach ☐ Rectum
☐ Other ______________________

Medications

____
____
____
____
____

Notes

Daily Tracking

DATE:

S M T W T F S

Fluid Tracker 8 oz 8 oz 8 oz 8 oz 8 oz 8 oz 8 oz 8 oz

Meal Tracking

Time	Meal	Pain Scale 0-5 0= No pain 5= Severe
BREAKFAST		
LUNCH		
DINNER		
SNACKS		

Bowel Activity

Normal	Very Hard	Abnormalities
		☐ Blood ☐ Mucus ☐ Other ______
		☐ Blood ☐ Mucus ☐ Other ______
		☐ Blood ☐ Mucus ☐ Other ______
		☐ Blood ☐ Mucus ☐ Other ______
	More?	

Other Symptoms

☐ Bloating ☐ Fatigue
☐ Nausea ☐ Flatulence
☐ Vomiting
☐ Other ______________________

Stress Level

Sleep

Energy Level

Activity Level

Pain Location (If Applicable)

☐ Abdomen ☐ Joints
☐ Stomach ☐ Rectum
☐ Other ______________________

Medications

____
____
____
____
____

Notes

Daily Tracking

DATE:

S M T W T F S

Fluid Tracker 8 oz 8 oz 8 oz 8 oz 8 oz 8 oz 8 oz 8 oz

Meal Tracking

Time	Meal	Pain Scale 0-5 0= No pain 5= Severe
BREAKFAST		
LUNCH		
DINNER		
SNACKS		

Bowel Activity

Normal	Very Hard	Abnormalities
		☐ Blood ☐ Mucus ☐ Other ______
		☐ Blood ☐ Mucus ☐ Other ______
		☐ Blood ☐ Mucus ☐ Other ______
		☐ Blood ☐ Mucus ☐ Other ______
	More?	

Pain Location (If Applicable)

☐ Abdomen ☐ Joints
☐ Stomach ☐ Rectum
☐ Other ______________

Notes

Other Symptoms

☐ Bloating ☐ Fatigue
☐ Nausea ☐ Flatulence
☐ Vomiting
☐ Other ______________

Stress Level

Sleep

Energy Level

Activity Level

Medications

____
____
____
____
____

Daily Tracking

DATE:

S M T W T F S

Fluid Tracker 8 oz 8 oz 8 oz 8 oz 8 oz 8 oz 8 oz 8 oz

Meal Tracking

Time	Meal	Pain Scale 0-5 0= No pain 5= Severe
BREAKFAST		
LUNCH		
DINNER		
SNACKS		

Bowel Activity

Normal	Very Hard	Abnormalities
		☐ Blood ☐ Mucus ☐ Other ______
		☐ Blood ☐ Mucus ☐ Other ______
		☐ Blood ☐ Mucus ☐ Other ______
		☐ Blood ☐ Mucus ☐ Other ______
	More?	

Other Symptoms

- ☐ Bloating
- ☐ Fatigue
- ☐ Nausea
- ☐ Flatulence
- ☐ Vomiting
- ☐ Other ______

Stress Level

Sleep

Energy Level

Activity Level

Pain Location (If Applicable)

- ☐ Abdomen
- ☐ Joints
- ☐ Stomach
- ☐ Rectum
- ☐ Other ______

Medications

Notes

Daily Tracking

DATE:

S M T W T F S

Fluid Tracker: 8 oz | 8 oz | 8 oz | 8 oz | 8 oz | 8 oz | 8 oz | 8 oz

Meal Tracking

Time	Meal	Pain Scale 0-5 0= No pain 5= Severe
BREAKFAST		
LUNCH		
DINNER		
SNACKS		

Bowel Activity

Normal	Very Hard	Abnormalities
		☐ Blood ☐ Mucus ☐ Other ______
		☐ Blood ☐ Mucus ☐ Other ______
		☐ Blood ☐ Mucus ☐ Other ______
		☐ Blood ☐ Mucus ☐ Other ______
	More?	

Pain Location (If Applicable)

☐ Abdomen ☐ Joints
☐ Stomach ☐ Rectum
☐ Other ______________________

Notes

Other Symptoms

☐ Bloating ☐ Fatigue
☐ Nausea ☐ Flatulence
☐ Vomiting
☐ Other ______________________

Stress Level

Sleep

Energy Level

Activity Level

Medications

____
____
____
____
____

Daily Tracking

DATE:

S M T W T F S

Fluid Tracker 8 oz 8 oz 8 oz 8 oz 8 oz 8 oz 8 oz 8 oz

Meal Tracking

Time	Meal	Pain Scale 0-5 0= No pain 5= Severe
BREAKFAST		
LUNCH		
DINNER		
SNACKS		

Bowel Activity

Normal	Very Hard	Abnormalities
		☐ Blood ☐ Mucus ☐ Other ______
		☐ Blood ☐ Mucus ☐ Other ______
		☐ Blood ☐ Mucus ☐ Other ______
		☐ Blood ☐ Mucus ☐ Other ______
	More?	

Other Symptoms

☐ Bloating ☐ Fatigue
☐ Nausea ☐ Flatulence
☐ Vomiting
☐ Other ______________________

Stress Level

Sleep

Energy Level

Activity Level

Pain Location (If Applicable)

☐ Abdomen ☐ Joints
☐ Stomach ☐ Rectum
☐ Other ______________________

Medications

____
____
____
____
____

Notes

Daily Tracking

DATE:

S M T W T F S

Fluid Tracker 8 oz 8 oz 8 oz 8 oz 8 oz 8 oz 8 oz 8 oz

Meal Tracking

Time	Meal	Pain Scale 0-5 0= No pain 5= Severe
BREAKFAST		
LUNCH		
DINNER		
SNACKS		

Bowel Activity

Normal	Very Hard	Abnormalities
		☐ Blood ☐ Mucus ☐ Other ______
		☐ Blood ☐ Mucus ☐ Other ______
		☐ Blood ☐ Mucus ☐ Other ______
		☐ Blood ☐ Mucus ☐ Other ______
	More?	

Other Symptoms

☐ Bloating ☐ Fatigue
☐ Nausea ☐ Flatulence
☐ Vomiting
☐ Other ______________________

Stress Level

Sleep

Energy Level

Activity Leve

Pain Location (If Applicable)

☐ Abdomen ☐ Joints
☐ Stomach ☐ Rectum
☐ Other ______________________

Medications

____

____

____

____

____

Notes

Weekly Reflections

What was the best thing that happened this week?

What was the hardest thing that happened this week?

What helped you the most this week?

What gave you hope this week?

What's one small win you can celebrate?

Was there something that eased your stress?

Overall, this week I felt

☐ A little better ☐ A lot better ☐ A little worse ☐ A lot worse

☐ About the same

Next week I want to:

____

____

____

____

Healing takes time. Let yourself grow at your own pace.

Daily Tracking

DATE:

S M T W T F S

Fluid Tracker: 8 oz | 8 oz | 8 oz | 8 oz | 8 oz | 8 oz | 8 oz | 8 oz

Meal Tracking

Time	Meal	Pain Scale 0-5 0= No pain 5= Severe
BREAKFAST		
LUNCH		
DINNER		
SNACKS		

Bowel Activity

Normal	Very Hard	Abnormalities
		☐ Blood ☐ Mucus ☐ Other ______
		☐ Blood ☐ Mucus ☐ Other ______
		☐ Blood ☐ Mucus ☐ Other ______
		☐ Blood ☐ Mucus ☐ Other ______
	More?	

Other Symptoms

☐ Bloating ☐ Fatigue
☐ Nausea ☐ Flatulence
☐ Vomiting
☐ Other ______________________

Stress Level

Sleep

Energy Level

Activity Level

Pain Location (If Applicable)

☐ Abdomen ☐ Joints
☐ Stomach ☐ Rectum
☐ Other ______________________

Medications

____
____
____
____
____

Notes

Daily Tracking

DATE:

S M T W T F S

Meal Tracking

Fluid Tracker: 8 oz | 8 oz | 8 oz | 8 oz | 8 oz | 8 oz | 8 oz | 8 oz

Time	Meal	Pain Scale 0-5 0= No pain 5= Severe
BREAKFAST		
LUNCH		
DINNER		
SNACKS		

Bowel Activity

Normal	Very Hard	Abnormalities
		☐ Blood ☐ Mucus ☐ Other ______
		☐ Blood ☐ Mucus ☐ Other ______
		☐ Blood ☐ Mucus ☐ Other ______
		☐ Blood ☐ Mucus ☐ Other ______
	More?	

Other Symptoms

☐ Bloating ☐ Fatigue
☐ Nausea ☐ Flatulence
☐ Vomiting
☐ Other ______________________

Stress Level

Sleep

Energy Level

Activity Level

Pain Location (If Applicable)

☐ Abdomen ☐ Joints
☐ Stomach ☐ Rectum
☐ Other ______________________

Notes

Medications

____
____
____
____
____

Daily Tracking

DATE:

S M T W T F S

Fluid Tracker 8 oz 8 oz 8 oz 8 oz 8 oz 8 oz 8 oz 8 oz

Meal Tracking

Time	Meal	Pain Scale 0-5 0= No pain 5= Severe
BREAKFAST		
LUNCH		
DINNER		
SNACKS		

Bowel Activity

Normal	Very Hard	Abnormalities
		☐ Blood ☐ Mucus ☐ Other ______
		☐ Blood ☐ Mucus ☐ Other ______
		☐ Blood ☐ Mucus ☐ Other ______
		☐ Blood ☐ Mucus ☐ Other ______
	More?	

Other Symptoms

☐ Bloating ☐ Fatigue
☐ Nausea ☐ Flatulence
☐ Vomiting
☐ Other ______________________

Stress Level

Sleep

Energy Level

Activity Level

Pain Location (If Applicable)

☐ Abdomen ☐ Joints
☐ Stomach ☐ Rectum
☐ Other ______________________

Notes

Medications

____
____
____
____
____

Daily Tracking

DATE:

S M T W T F S

Fluid Tracker: 8 oz 8 oz 8 oz 8 oz 8 oz 8 oz 8 oz 8 oz

Meal Tracking

Time	Meal	Pain Scale 0-5 0= No pain 5= Severe
BREAKFAST		
LUNCH		
DINNER		
SNACKS		

Bowel Activity

Normal	Very Hard	Abnormalities
		☐ Blood ☐ Mucus ☐ Other ______
		☐ Blood ☐ Mucus ☐ Other ______
		☐ Blood ☐ Mucus ☐ Other ______
		☐ Blood ☐ Mucus ☐ Other ______
	More?	

Pain Location (If Applicable)

☐ Abdomen ☐ Joints
☐ Stomach ☐ Rectum
☐ Other ______________________

Notes

Other Symptoms

☐ Bloating ☐ Fatigue
☐ Nausea ☐ Flatulence
☐ Vomiting
☐ Other ______________________

Stress Level

Sleep

Energy Level

Activity Level

Medications

____

____

____

____

____

Daily Tracking

DATE:

S M T W T F S

Fluid Tracker 8 oz 8 oz 8 oz 8 oz 8 oz 8 oz 8 oz 8 oz

Meal Tracking

Time	Meal	Pain Scale 0-5 0= No pain 5= Severe
BREAKFAST		
LUNCH		
DINNER		
SNACKS		

Bowel Activity

Normal	Very Hard	Abnormalities
		☐ Blood ☐ Mucus ☐ Other ______
		☐ Blood ☐ Mucus ☐ Other ______
		☐ Blood ☐ Mucus ☐ Other ______
		☐ Blood ☐ Mucus ☐ Other ______
	More?	

Other Symptoms

☐ Bloating ☐ Fatigue
☐ Nausea ☐ Flatulence
☐ Vomiting
☐ Other ______

Stress Level

Sleep

Energy Level

Activity Level

Pain Location (If Applicable)

☐ Abdomen ☐ Joints
☐ Stomach ☐ Rectum
☐ Other ______

Medications

______
______
______
______
______

Notes

Daily Tracking

DATE:

S M T W T F S

Fluid Tracker: 8 oz | 8 oz | 8 oz | 8 oz | 8 oz | 8 oz | 8 oz | 8 oz

Meal Tracking

Time	Meal	Pain Scale 0-5 0= No pain 5= Severe
BREAKFAST		
LUNCH		
DINNER		
SNACKS		

Bowel Activity

Normal	Very Hard	Abnormalities
		☐ Blood ☐ Mucus ☐ Other
		☐ Blood ☐ Mucus ☐ Other
		☐ Blood ☐ Mucus ☐ Other
		☐ Blood ☐ Mucus ☐ Other
	More?	

Other Symptoms

☐ Bloating ☐ Fatigue
☐ Nausea ☐ Flatulence
☐ Vomiting
☐ Other ________________

Stress Level

Sleep

Energy Level

Activity Level

Pain Location (If Applicable)

☐ Abdomen ☐ Joints
☐ Stomach ☐ Rectum
☐ Other ________________

Medications

Notes

Daily Tracking

DATE:

S M T W T F S

Fluid Tracker: 8 oz | 8 oz | 8 oz | 8 oz | 8 oz | 8 oz | 8 oz | 8 oz

Meal Tracking

Time	Meal	Pain Scale 0-5 0= No pain 5= Severe
BREAKFAST		
LUNCH		
DINNER		
SNACKS		

Bowel Activity

Normal	Very Hard	Abnormalities
		☐ Blood ☐ Mucus ☐ Other ______
		☐ Blood ☐ Mucus ☐ Other ______
		☐ Blood ☐ Mucus ☐ Other ______
		☐ Blood ☐ Mucus ☐ Other ______
	More?	

Other Symptoms

- ☐ Bloating
- ☐ Fatigue
- ☐ Nausea
- ☐ Flatulence
- ☐ Vomiting
- ☐ Other ______________________

Stress Level

Sleep

Energy Level

Activity Leve

Pain Location (If Applicable)

- ☐ Abdomen
- ☐ Joints
- ☐ Stomach
- ☐ Rectum
- ☐ Other ______________________

Notes

Medications

____

____

____

____

____

Weekly Reflections

What was the best thing that happened this week?

What was the hardest thing that happened this week?

What helped you the most this week?

What gave you hope this week?

What's one small win you can celebrate?

Was there something that eased your stress?

Overall, this week I felt

☐ A little better ☐ A lot better ☐ A little worse ☐ A lot worse

☐ About the same

Next week I want to:

____

____

____

____

A tough day doesn't undo your progress. Tomorrow is another page waiting for you.

Daily Tracking

DATE:

S M T W T F S

Fluid Tracker: 8 oz | 8 oz | 8 oz | 8 oz | 8 oz | 8 oz | 8 oz | 8 oz

Meal Tracking

Time	Meal	Pain Scale 0-5 0= No pain 5= Severe
BREAKFAST		
LUNCH		
DINNER		
SNACKS		

Bowel Activity

Normal	Very Hard	Abnormalities
		☐ Blood ☐ Mucus ☐ Other ______
		☐ Blood ☐ Mucus ☐ Other ______
		☐ Blood ☐ Mucus ☐ Other ______
		☐ Blood ☐ Mucus ☐ Other ______
	More?	

Other Symptoms

- ☐ Bloating
- ☐ Fatigue
- ☐ Nausea
- ☐ Flatulence
- ☐ Vomiting
- ☐ Other ______________________

Stress Level

Sleep

Energy Level

Activity Level

Pain Location (If Applicable)

- ☐ Abdomen
- ☐ Joints
- ☐ Stomach
- ☐ Rectum
- ☐ Other ______________________

Notes

Medications

____

____

____

____

____

Daily Tracking

DATE:

S M T W T F S

Meal Tracking

Fluid Tracker: 8 oz | 8 oz | 8 oz | 8 oz | 8 oz | 8 oz | 8 oz | 8 oz

Time	Meal	Pain Scale 0-5 0= No pain 5= Severe
BREAKFAST		
LUNCH		
DINNER		
SNACKS		

Bowel Activity

Normal	Very Hard	Abnormalities
		☐ Blood ☐ Mucus ☐ Other ____
		☐ Blood ☐ Mucus ☐ Other ____
		☐ Blood ☐ Mucus ☐ Other ____
		☐ Blood ☐ Mucus ☐ Other ____
	More?	

Other Symptoms

☐ Bloating ☐ Fatigue
☐ Nausea ☐ Flatulence
☐ Vomiting
☐ Other ____________________

Stress Level

Sleep

Energy Level

Activity Level

Pain Location (If Applicable)

☐ Abdomen ☐ Joints
☐ Stomach ☐ Rectum
☐ Other ____________________

Medications

____
____
____
____
____

Notes

Daily Tracking

DATE:

S M T W T F S

Meal Tracking

Fluid Tracker: 8 oz | 8 oz | 8 oz | 8 oz | 8 oz | 8 oz | 8 oz | 8 oz

Time	Meal	Pain Scale 0-5 0= No pain 5= Severe
BREAKFAST		
LUNCH		
DINNER		
SNACKS		

Bowel Activity

Normal	Very Hard	Abnormalities
		☐ Blood ☐ Mucus ☐ Other ____
		☐ Blood ☐ Mucus ☐ Other ____
		☐ Blood ☐ Mucus ☐ Other ____
		☐ Blood ☐ Mucus ☐ Other ____
	More?	

Other Symptoms

☐ Bloating ☐ Fatigue
☐ Nausea ☐ Flatulence
☐ Vomiting
☐ Other ____________________

Stress Level

Sleep

Energy Level

Activity Level

Pain Location (If Applicable)

☐ Abdomen ☐ Joints
☐ Stomach ☐ Rectum
☐ Other ____________________

Medications

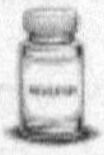

____

____

____

____

____

Notes

Daily Tracking

DATE:

S M T W T F S

Fluid Tracker 8 oz 8 oz 8 oz 8 oz 8 oz 8 oz 8 oz 8 oz

Meal Tracking

Time	Meal	Pain Scale 0-5 0= No pain 5= Severe
BREAKFAST		
LUNCH		
DINNER		
SNACKS		

Bowel Activity

Normal	Very Hard	Abnormalities
		☐ Blood ☐ Mucus ☐ Other
		☐ Blood ☐ Mucus ☐ Other
		☐ Blood ☐ Mucus ☐ Other
		☐ Blood ☐ Mucus ☐ Other
	More?	

Other Symptoms

- ☐ Bloating
- ☐ Fatigue
- ☐ Nausea
- ☐ Flatulence
- ☐ Vomiting
- ☐ Other ________________

Stress Level

Sleep

Energy Level

Activity Level

Pain Location (If Applicable)

- ☐ Abdomen
- ☐ Joints
- ☐ Stomach
- ☐ Rectum
- ☐ Other ________________

Notes

Medications

Daily Tracking

DATE:

S M T W T F S

Fluid Tracker: 8 oz | 8 oz | 8 oz | 8 oz | 8 oz | 8 oz | 8 oz | 8 oz

Meal Tracking

Time	Meal	Pain Scale 0-5 0= No pain 5= Severe
BREAKFAST		
LUNCH		
DINNER		
SNACKS		

Bowel Activity

Normal	Very Hard	Abnormalities
		☐ Blood ☐ Mucus ☐ Other ______
		☐ Blood ☐ Mucus ☐ Other ______
		☐ Blood ☐ Mucus ☐ Other ______
		☐ Blood ☐ Mucus ☐ Other ______
	More?	

Other Symptoms

☐ Bloating ☐ Fatigue
☐ Nausea ☐ Flatulence
☐ Vomiting
☐ Other ______________________

Stress Level

Sleep

Energy Level

Activity Level

Pain Location (If Applicable)

☐ Abdomen ☐ Joints
☐ Stomach ☐ Rectum
☐ Other ______________________

Medications

____
____
____
____
____

Notes

Daily Tracking

DATE: ____________________

S M T W T F S

Fluid Tracker 8 oz | 8 oz | 8 oz | 8 oz | 8 oz | 8 oz | 8 oz | 8 oz

Meal Tracking

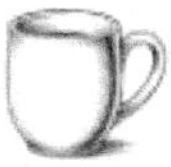

Time	Meal	Pain Scale 0-5 0= No pain 5= Severe
BREAKFAST		
LUNCH		
DINNER		
SNACKS		

Bowel Activity

Normal	Very Hard	Abnormalities
		☐ Blood ☐ Mucus ☐ Other ________
		☐ Blood ☐ Mucus ☐ Other ________
		☐ Blood ☐ Mucus ☐ Other ________
		☐ Blood ☐ Mucus ☐ Other ________
	More?	

Other Symptoms

☐ Bloating ☐ Fatigue
☐ Nausea ☐ Flatulence
☐ Vomiting
☐ Other ____________________

Stress Level

Sleep

Energy Level

Activity Level

Pain Location (If Applicable)

☐ Abdomen ☐ Joints
☐ Stomach ☐ Rectum
☐ Other ____________________

Notes

Medications

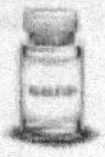

____
____
____
____
____

Daily Tracking

DATE:	S M T W T F S

Fluid Tracker 8 oz | 8 oz | 8 oz | 8 oz | 8 oz | 8 oz | 8 oz | 8 oz

Meal Tracking

Time	Meal	Pain Scale 0-5 0= No pain 5= Severe
BREAKFAST		
LUNCH		
DINNER		
SNACKS		

Bowel Activity

Normal	Very Hard	Abnormalities
		☐ Blood ☐ Mucus ☐ Other ______
		☐ Blood ☐ Mucus ☐ Other ______
		☐ Blood ☐ Mucus ☐ Other ______
		☐ Blood ☐ Mucus ☐ Other ______
	More?	

Other Symptoms

- ☐ Bloating
- ☐ Fatigue
- ☐ Nausea
- ☐ Flatulence
- ☐ Vomiting
- ☐ Other ______________________

Pain Location (If Applicable)

- ☐ Abdomen
- ☐ Joints
- ☐ Stomach
- ☐ Rectum
- ☐ Other ______________________

Stress Level

Sleep

Energy Level

Activity Level

Medications

____

____

____

____

____

Notes

Weekly Reflections

What was the best thing that happened this week?

What was the hardest thing that happened this week?

What helped you the most this week?

What gave you hope this week?

What's one small win you can celebrate?

Was there something that eased your stress?

Overall, this week I felt

☐ A little better ☐ A lot better ☐ A little worse ☐ A lot worse
☐ About the same

Next week I want to:

____

____

____

____

Celebrate your wins, even the smallest ones—they build into something greater.

Monthly Thoughts

This page is your space to step back and see the bigger picture. Each month brings its own challenges and small victories—use this space to notice patterns, celebrate progress, and reflect on what your body and mind are teaching you. These notes can guide you forward with greater clarity and self-compassion.

This Month I Noticed...

(Write down patterns in your symptoms, energy, or mood.)

Biggest Challenge: ____

____

Brightest Moment: ____

____

Triggers I Noticed: ____

____

Things That Helped: ____

____

Medication / Treatment Notes: (Any changes, side effects, or adjustments.) ______________________________

____

____

Self-Care Check-In

How well I cared for myself this month: ______________________

____

Looking Forward

Next month I want to focus on: ______________________________

____

____

Symptom Overview

Good Days: ________ Mild Days: ________ Flare Days: ________

Your progress is not erased by setbacks—it's carried within you.

Daily Tracking

DATE:

S M T W T F S

Fluid Tracker: 8 oz | 8 oz | 8 oz | 8 oz | 8 oz | 8 oz | 8 oz | 8 oz

Meal Tracking

Time	Meal	Pain Scale 0-5 0= No pain 5= Severe
BREAKFAST		
LUNCH		
DINNER		
SNACKS		

Bowel Activity

Normal	Very Hard	Abnormalities
		☐ Blood ☐ Mucus ☐ Other ______
		☐ Blood ☐ Mucus ☐ Other ______
		☐ Blood ☐ Mucus ☐ Other ______
		☐ Blood ☐ Mucus ☐ Other ______
	More?	

Other Symptoms

- ☐ Bloating
- ☐ Fatigue
- ☐ Nausea
- ☐ Flatulence
- ☐ Vomiting
- ☐ Other ______________________

Pain Location (If Applicable)

- ☐ Abdomen
- ☐ Joints
- ☐ Stomach
- ☐ Rectum
- ☐ Other ______________________

Stress Level

Sleep

Energy Level

Activity Level

Medications

____

____

____

____

____

Notes

Daily Tracking

DATE:

S M T W T F S

Fluid Tracker: 8 oz | 8 oz | 8 oz | 8 oz | 8 oz | 8 oz | 8 oz | 8 oz

Meal Tracking

Time	Meal	Pain Scale 0-5 0= No pain 5= Severe
BREAKFAST		
LUNCH		
DINNER		
SNACKS		

Bowel Activity

Normal	Very Hard	Abnormalities
		☐ Blood ☐ Mucus ☐ Other ______
		☐ Blood ☐ Mucus ☐ Other ______
		☐ Blood ☐ Mucus ☐ Other ______
		☐ Blood ☐ Mucus ☐ Other ______
	More?	

Other Symptoms

☐ Bloating ☐ Fatigue
☐ Nausea ☐ Flatulence
☐ Vomiting
☐ Other ______________________

Stress Level

Sleep

Energy Level

Activity Level

Pain Location (If Applicable)

☐ Abdomen ☐ Joints
☐ Stomach ☐ Rectum
☐ Other ______________________

Medications

____
____
____
____
____

Notes

Daily Tracking

DATE:

S M T W T F S

Fluid Tracker 8 oz 8 oz 8 oz 8 oz 8 oz 8 oz 8 oz 8 oz

Meal Tracking

Time	Meal	Pain Scale 0-5 0= No pain 5= Severe
BREAKFAST		
LUNCH		
DINNER		
SNACKS		

Bowel Activity

Normal	Very Hard	Abnormalities
		☐ Blood ☐ Mucus ☐ Other ____
		☐ Blood ☐ Mucus ☐ Other ____
		☐ Blood ☐ Mucus ☐ Other ____
		☐ Blood ☐ Mucus ☐ Other ____
	More?	

Other Symptoms

☐ Bloating ☐ Fatigue
☐ Nausea ☐ Flatulence
☐ Vomiting
☐ Other ____________________

Stress Level

Sleep

Energy Level

Activity Level

Pain Location (If Applicable)

☐ Abdomen ☐ Joints
☐ Stomach ☐ Rectum
☐ Other ____________________

Medications

____
____
____
____
____

Notes

Daily Tracking

DATE:

S M T W T F S

Fluid Tracker 8 oz 8 oz 8 oz 8 oz 8 oz 8 oz 8 oz 8 oz

Meal Tracking

Time	Meal	Pain Scale 0-5 0= No pain 5= Severe
BREAKFAST		
LUNCH		
DINNER		
SNACKS		

Bowel Activity

Normal	Very Hard	Abnormalities
		☐ Blood ☐ Mucus ☐ Other ______
		☐ Blood ☐ Mucus ☐ Other ______
		☐ Blood ☐ Mucus ☐ Other ______
		☐ Blood ☐ Mucus ☐ Other ______
	More?	

Other Symptoms

- ☐ Bloating
- ☐ Fatigue
- ☐ Nausea
- ☐ Flatulence
- ☐ Vomiting
- ☐ Other ______________________

Stress Level

Sleep

Energy Level

Activity Level

Pain Location (If Applicable)

- ☐ Abdomen
- ☐ Joints
- ☐ Stomach
- ☐ Rectum
- ☐ Other ______________________

Medications

____

____

____

____

____

Notes

Daily Tracking

DATE:

S M T W T F S

Fluid Tracker: 8 oz | 8 oz | 8 oz | 8 oz | 8 oz | 8 oz | 8 oz | 8 oz

Meal Tracking

Time	Meal	Pain Scale 0-5 0= No pain 5= Severe
BREAKFAST		
LUNCH		
DINNER		
SNACKS		

Bowel Activity

Normal	Very Hard	Abnormalities
		☐ Blood ☐ Mucus ☐ Other ______
		☐ Blood ☐ Mucus ☐ Other ______
		☐ Blood ☐ Mucus ☐ Other ______
		☐ Blood ☐ Mucus ☐ Other ______
	More?	

Other Symptoms

☐ Bloating ☐ Fatigue
☐ Nausea ☐ Flatulence
☐ Vomiting
☐ Other ______________________

Stress Level

Sleep

Energy Level

Activity Level

Pain Location (If Applicable)

☐ Abdomen ☐ Joints
☐ Stomach ☐ Rectum
☐ Other ______________________

Medications

____
____
____
____
____

Notes

Daily Tracking

DATE:

S M T W T F S

Fluid Tracker 8 oz 8 oz 8 oz 8 oz 8 oz 8 oz 8 oz 8 oz

Meal Tracking

Time	Meal	Pain Scale 0-5 0= No pain 5= Severe
BREAKFAST		
LUNCH		
DINNER		
SNACKS		

Bowel Activity

Normal	Very Hard	Abnormalities
		☐ Blood ☐ Mucus ☐ Other ______
		☐ Blood ☐ Mucus ☐ Other ______
		☐ Blood ☐ Mucus ☐ Other ______
		☐ Blood ☐ Mucus ☐ Other ______
	More?	

Other Symptoms

☐ Bloating ☐ Fatigue
☐ Nausea ☐ Flatulence
☐ Vomiting
☐ Other ______________________

Stress Level

Sleep

Energy Level

Activity Level

Pain Location (If Applicable)

☐ Abdomen ☐ Joints
☐ Stomach ☐ Rectum
☐ Other ______________________

Notes

Medications

____
____
____
____
____

Daily Tracking

DATE:

S M T W T F S

Fluid Tracker 8 oz 8 oz 8 oz 8 oz 8 oz 8 oz 8 oz 8 oz

Meal Tracking

Time	Meal	Pain Scale 0-5 0= No pain 5= Severe
BREAKFAST		
LUNCH		
DINNER		
SNACKS		

Bowel Activity

Normal	Very Hard	Abnormalities
		☐ Blood ☐ Mucus ☐ Other ______
		☐ Blood ☐ Mucus ☐ Other ______
		☐ Blood ☐ Mucus ☐ Other ______
		☐ Blood ☐ Mucus ☐ Other ______
	More?	

Other Symptoms

☐ Bloating ☐ Fatigue
☐ Nausea ☐ Flatulence
☐ Vomiting
☐ Other ______________________

Stress Level

Sleep

Energy Level

Activity Level

Pain Location (If Applicable)

☐ Abdomen ☐ Joints
☐ Stomach ☐ Rectum
☐ Other ______________________

Medications

____
____
____
____
____

Notes

Weekly Reflections

What was the best thing that happened this week?

What was the hardest thing that happened this week?

What helped you the most this week?

What gave you hope this week?

What's one small win you can celebrate?

Was there something that eased your stress?

Overall, this week I felt

☐ A little better ☐ A lot better ☐ A little worse ☐ A lot worse

☐ About the same

Next week I want to:

____

____

____

____

Reflection isn't about perfection. It's about noticing, learning, and honoring yourself.

Daily Tracking

DATE:

S M T W T F S

Meal Tracking

Fluid Tracker: 8 oz 8 oz 8 oz 8 oz 8 oz 8 oz 8 oz 8 oz

Time	Meal	Pain Scale 0-5 0= No pain 5= Severe
BREAKFAST		
LUNCH		
DINNER		
SNACKS		

Bowel Activity

Normal	Very Hard	Abnormalities
		☐ Blood ☐ Mucus ☐ Other ______
		☐ Blood ☐ Mucus ☐ Other ______
		☐ Blood ☐ Mucus ☐ Other ______
		☐ Blood ☐ Mucus ☐ Other ______
	More?	

Other Symptoms

☐ Bloating ☐ Fatigue
☐ Nausea ☐ Flatulence
☐ Vomiting
☐ Other ______________________

Stress Level

Sleep

Energy Level

Activity Level

Pain Location (If Applicable)

☐ Abdomen ☐ Joints
☐ Stomach ☐ Rectum
☐ Other ______________________

Medications

____
____
____
____
____

Notes

Daily Tracking

DATE: ____________________ (S) (M) (T) (W) (T) (F) (S)

Fluid Tracker 8 oz 8 oz 8 oz 8 oz 8 oz 8 oz 8 oz 8 oz

Meal Tracking

Time	Meal	Pain Scale 0-5 0= No pain 5= Severe
BREAKFAST		
LUNCH		
DINNER		
SNACKS		

Bowel Activity

Normal	Very Hard	Abnormalities
		☐ Blood ☐ Mucus ☐ Other ______
		☐ Blood ☐ Mucus ☐ Other ______
		☐ Blood ☐ Mucus ☐ Other ______
		☐ Blood ☐ Mucus ☐ Other ______
	More?	

Other Symptoms

☐ Bloating ☐ Fatigue
☐ Nausea ☐ Flatulence
☐ Vomiting
☐ Other ____________________

Stress Level

Sleep

Energy Level

Activity Level

Pain Location (If Applicable)

☐ Abdomen ☐ Joints
☐ Stomach ☐ Rectum
☐ Other ____________________

Medications

____
____
____
____
____

Notes

Daily Tracking

DATE:

S M T W T F S

Fluid Tracker 8 oz 8 oz 8 oz 8 oz 8 oz 8 oz 8 oz 8 oz

Meal Tracking

Time	Meal	Pain Scale 0-5 0= No pain 5= Severe
BREAKFAST		
LUNCH		
DINNER		
SNACKS		

Bowel Activity

Normal	Very Hard	Abnormalities
		☐ Blood ☐ Mucus ☐ Other ______
		☐ Blood ☐ Mucus ☐ Other ______
		☐ Blood ☐ Mucus ☐ Other ______
		☐ Blood ☐ Mucus ☐ Other ______
	More?	

Other Symptoms

☐ Bloating ☐ Fatigue
☐ Nausea ☐ Flatulence
☐ Vomiting
☐ Other ______________________

Stress Level

Sleep

Energy Level

Activity Level

Pain Location (If Applicable)

☐ Abdomen ☐ Joints
☐ Stomach ☐ Rectum
☐ Other ______________________

Medications

____
____
____
____
____

Notes

Daily Tracking

DATE:

S M T W T F S

Fluid Tracker: 8 oz | 8 oz | 8 oz | 8 oz | 8 oz | 8 oz | 8 oz | 8 oz

Meal Tracking

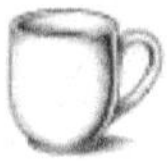

Time	Meal	Pain Scale 0-5 0= No pain 5= Severe
BREAKFAST		
LUNCH		
DINNER		
SNACKS		

Bowel Activity

Normal	Very Hard	Abnormalities
		☐ Blood ☐ Mucus ☐ Other ______
		☐ Blood ☐ Mucus ☐ Other ______
		☐ Blood ☐ Mucus ☐ Other ______
		☐ Blood ☐ Mucus ☐ Other ______
	More?	

Other Symptoms

- ☐ Bloating
- ☐ Fatigue
- ☐ Nausea
- ☐ Flatulence
- ☐ Vomiting
- ☐ Other ______________________

Stress Level

Sleep

Energy Level

Activity Level

Pain Location (If Applicable)

- ☐ Abdomen
- ☐ Joints
- ☐ Stomach
- ☐ Rectum
- ☐ Other ______________________

Medications

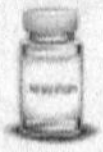

____

____

____

____

____

Notes

Daily Tracking

DATE:

S M T W T F S

Fluid Tracker: 8 oz | 8 oz | 8 oz | 8 oz | 8 oz | 8 oz | 8 oz | 8 oz

Meal Tracking

Time	Meal	Pain Scale 0-5 0= No pain 5= Severe
BREAKFAST		
LUNCH		
DINNER		
SNACKS		

Bowel Activity

Normal	Very Hard	Abnormalities
		☐ Blood ☐ Mucus ☐ Other ____
		☐ Blood ☐ Mucus ☐ Other ____
		☐ Blood ☐ Mucus ☐ Other ____
		☐ Blood ☐ Mucus ☐ Other ____
	More?	

Other Symptoms

- ☐ Bloating
- ☐ Fatigue
- ☐ Nausea
- ☐ Flatulence
- ☐ Vomiting
- ☐ Other ____________________

Stress Level

Sleep

Energy Level

Activity Level

Pain Location (If Applicable)

- ☐ Abdomen
- ☐ Joints
- ☐ Stomach
- ☐ Rectum
- ☐ Other ____________________

Medications

Notes

Daily Tracking

DATE:

S M T W T F S

Fluid Tracker 8 oz 8 oz 8 oz 8 oz 8 oz 8 oz 8 oz 8 oz

Meal Tracking

Time	Meal	Pain Scale 0-5 0= No pain 5= Severe
BREAKFAST		
LUNCH		
DINNER		
SNACKS		

Bowel Activity

Normal	Very Hard	Abnormalities
		☐ Blood ☐ Mucus ☐ Other ____
		☐ Blood ☐ Mucus ☐ Other ____
		☐ Blood ☐ Mucus ☐ Other ____
		☐ Blood ☐ Mucus ☐ Other ____
	More?	

Other Symptoms

☐ Bloating ☐ Fatigue
☐ Nausea ☐ Flatulence
☐ Vomiting
☐ Other ____________

Stress Level

Sleep

Energy Level

Activity Level

Pain Location (If Applicable)

☐ Abdomen ☐ Joints
☐ Stomach ☐ Rectum
☐ Other ____________

Medications

Notes

Daily Tracking

DATE:	S M T W T F S

Fluid Tracker: 8 oz | 8 oz | 8 oz | 8 oz | 8 oz | 8 oz | 8 oz | 8 oz

Meal Tracking

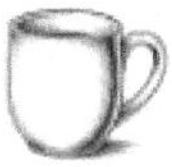

Time	Meal	Pain Scale 0-5 0= No pain 5= Severe
BREAKFAST		
LUNCH		
DINNER		
SNACKS		

Bowel Activity

Normal	Very Hard	Abnormalities
		☐ Blood ☐ Mucus ☐ Other ________
		☐ Blood ☐ Mucus ☐ Other ________
		☐ Blood ☐ Mucus ☐ Other ________
		☐ Blood ☐ Mucus ☐ Other ________
	More?	

Other Symptoms

☐ Bloating ☐ Fatigue
☐ Nausea ☐ Flatulence
☐ Vomiting
☐ Other ____________________

Stress Level

Sleep

Energy Level

Activity Level

Pain Location (If Applicable)

☐ Abdomen ☐ Joints
☐ Stomach ☐ Rectum
☐ Other ____________________

Medications

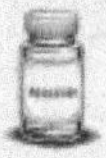

____
____
____
____
____

Notes

Weekly Reflections

What was the best thing that happened this week?

What was the hardest thing that happened this week?

What helped you the most this week?

What gave you hope this week?

What's one small win you can celebrate?

Was there something that eased your stress?

Overall, this week I felt

☐ A little better ☐ A lot better ☐ A little worse ☐ A lot worse

☐ About the same

Next week I want to:

____

____

____

____

Rest is productive. Your body heals best when you give it care and patience.

Daily Tracking

DATE:

S M T W T F S

Fluid Tracker 8 oz 8 oz 8 oz 8 oz 8 oz 8 oz 8 oz 8 oz

Meal Tracking

Time	Meal	Pain Scale 0-5 0= No pain 5= Severe
BREAKFAST		
LUNCH		
DINNER		
SNACKS		

Bowel Activity

Normal	Very Hard	Abnormalities
		☐ Blood ☐ Mucus ☐ Other ______
		☐ Blood ☐ Mucus ☐ Other ______
		☐ Blood ☐ Mucus ☐ Other ______
		☐ Blood ☐ Mucus ☐ Other ______
	More?	

Other Symptoms

☐ Bloating ☐ Fatigue
☐ Nausea ☐ Flatulence
☐ Vomiting
☐ Other ______________________

Stress Level

Sleep

Energy Level

Activity Level

Pain Location (If Applicable)

☐ Abdomen ☐ Joints
☐ Stomach ☐ Rectum
☐ Other ______________________

Medications

____
____
____
____
____

Notes

Daily Tracking

DATE:

S M T W T F S

Fluid Tracker 8 oz 8 oz 8 oz 8 oz 8 oz 8 oz 8 oz 8 oz

Meal Tracking

Time	Meal	Pain Scale 0-5 0= No pain 5= Severe
BREAKFAST		
LUNCH		
DINNER		
SNACKS		

Bowel Activity

Normal	Very Hard	Abnormalities
		☐ Blood ☐ Mucus ☐ Other ______
		☐ Blood ☐ Mucus ☐ Other ______
		☐ Blood ☐ Mucus ☐ Other ______
		☐ Blood ☐ Mucus ☐ Other ______
	More?	

Other Symptoms

☐ Bloating ☐ Fatigue
☐ Nausea ☐ Flatulence
☐ Vomiting
☐ Other ______________

Stress Level

Sleep

Energy Level

Activity Level

Pain Location (If Applicable)

☐ Abdomen ☐ Joints
☐ Stomach ☐ Rectum
☐ Other ______________

Notes

Medications

____

____

____

____

____

Daily Tracking

DATE:

S M T W T F S

Fluid Tracker: 8 oz | 8 oz | 8 oz | 8 oz | 8 oz | 8 oz | 8 oz | 8 oz

Meal Tracking

Time	Meal	Pain Scale 0-5 0= No pain 5= Severe
BREAKFAST		
LUNCH		
DINNER		
SNACKS		

Bowel Activity

Normal	Very Hard	Abnormalities
		☐ Blood ☐ Mucus ☐ Other ______
		☐ Blood ☐ Mucus ☐ Other ______
		☐ Blood ☐ Mucus ☐ Other ______
		☐ Blood ☐ Mucus ☐ Other ______
	More?	

Other Symptoms

☐ Bloating ☐ Fatigue
☐ Nausea ☐ Flatulence
☐ Vomiting
☐ Other ______________________

Stress Level

Sleep

Energy Level

Activity Level

Pain Location (If Applicable)

☐ Abdomen ☐ Joints
☐ Stomach ☐ Rectum
☐ Other ______________________

Medications

____
____
____
____
____

Notes

Daily Tracking

DATE:

S M T W T F S

Fluid Tracker: 8 oz 8 oz 8 oz 8 oz 8 oz 8 oz 8 oz 8 oz

Meal Tracking

Time	Meal	Pain Scale 0-5 0= No pain 5= Severe
BREAKFAST		
LUNCH		
DINNER		
SNACKS		

Bowel Activity

Normal	Very Hard	Abnormalities
		☐ Blood ☐ Mucus ☐ Other ______
		☐ Blood ☐ Mucus ☐ Other ______
		☐ Blood ☐ Mucus ☐ Other ______
		☐ Blood ☐ Mucus ☐ Other ______
	More?	

Other Symptoms

☐ Bloating ☐ Fatigue
☐ Nausea ☐ Flatulence
☐ Vomiting
☐ Other ______________________

Stress Level

Sleep

Energy Level

Activity Level

Pain Location (If Applicable)

☐ Abdomen ☐ Joints
☐ Stomach ☐ Rectum
☐ Other ______________________

Medications

____
____
____
____
____

Notes

Daily Tracking

DATE:

S M T W T F S

Fluid Tracker: 8 oz | 8 oz | 8 oz | 8 oz | 8 oz | 8 oz | 8 oz | 8 oz

Meal Tracking

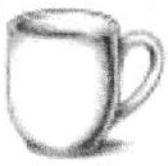

Time	Meal	Pain Scale 0-5 0= No pain 5= Severe
BREAKFAST		
LUNCH		
DINNER		
SNACKS		

Bowel Activity

Normal	Very Hard	Abnormalities
		☐ Blood ☐ Mucus ☐ Other ____
		☐ Blood ☐ Mucus ☐ Other ____
		☐ Blood ☐ Mucus ☐ Other ____
		☐ Blood ☐ Mucus ☐ Other ____
	More?	

Other Symptoms

☐ Bloating ☐ Fatigue
☐ Nausea ☐ Flatulence
☐ Vomiting
☐ Other ____________________

Stress Level

Sleep

Energy Level

Activity Level

Pain Location (If Applicable)

☐ Abdomen ☐ Joints
☐ Stomach ☐ Rectum
☐ Other ____________________

Medications

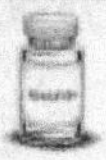

____
____
____
____
____

Notes

Daily Tracking

DATE:

S M T W T F S

Fluid Tracker: 8 oz | 8 oz | 8 oz | 8 oz | 8 oz | 8 oz | 8 oz | 8 oz

Meal Tracking

Time	Meal	Pain Scale 0-5 0= No pain 5= Severe
BREAKFAST		
LUNCH		
DINNER		
SNACKS		

Bowel Activity

Normal	Very Hard	Abnormalities
		☐ Blood ☐ Mucus ☐ Other ______
		☐ Blood ☐ Mucus ☐ Other ______
		☐ Blood ☐ Mucus ☐ Other ______
		☐ Blood ☐ Mucus ☐ Other ______
	More?	

Other Symptoms

- ☐ Bloating
- ☐ Fatigue
- ☐ Nausea
- ☐ Flatulence
- ☐ Vomiting
- ☐ Other ______________________

Stress Level

Sleep

Energy Level

Activity Level

Pain Location (If Applicable)

- ☐ Abdomen
- ☐ Joints
- ☐ Stomach
- ☐ Rectum
- ☐ Other ______________________

Medications

____

____

____

____

____

Notes

Daily Tracking

DATE:	S M T W T F S

Fluid Tracker: 8 oz | 8 oz | 8 oz | 8 oz | 8 oz | 8 oz | 8 oz | 8 oz

Meal Tracking

Time	Meal	Pain Scale 0-5 0= No pain 5= Severe
BREAKFAST		
LUNCH		
DINNER		
SNACKS		

Bowel Activity

Normal	Very Hard	Abnormalities
		☐ Blood ☐ Mucus ☐ Other ________
		☐ Blood ☐ Mucus ☐ Other ________
		☐ Blood ☐ Mucus ☐ Other ________
		☐ Blood ☐ Mucus ☐ Other ________
	More?	

Other Symptoms

- ☐ Bloating
- ☐ Fatigue
- ☐ Nausea
- ☐ Flatulence
- ☐ Vomiting
- ☐ Other ____________________

Stress Level

Sleep

Energy Level

Activity Level

Pain Location (If Applicable)

- ☐ Abdomen
- ☐ Joints
- ☐ Stomach
- ☐ Rectum
- ☐ Other ____________________

Medications

____

____

____

____

____

Notes

Weekly Reflections

What was the best thing that happened this week?

What was the hardest thing that happened this week?

What helped you the most this week?

What gave you hope this week?

What's one small win you can celebrate?

Was there something that eased your stress?

Overall, this week I felt

- ☐ A little better
- ☐ A lot better
- ☐ A little worse
- ☐ A lot worse
- ☐ About the same

Next week I want to:

____

____

____

____

Your voice matters. These pages are a safe space to let it be heard.

Daily Tracking

DATE:

S M T W T F S

Fluid Tracker: 8 oz | 8 oz | 8 oz | 8 oz | 8 oz | 8 oz | 8 oz | 8 oz

Meal Tracking

Time	Meal	Pain Scale 0-5 0= No pain 5= Severe
BREAKFAST		
LUNCH		
DINNER		
SNACKS		

Bowel Activity

Normal	Very Hard	Abnormalities
		☐ Blood ☐ Mucus ☐ Other ______
		☐ Blood ☐ Mucus ☐ Other ______
		☐ Blood ☐ Mucus ☐ Other ______
		☐ Blood ☐ Mucus ☐ Other ______
	More?	

Other Symptoms

☐ Bloating ☐ Fatigue
☐ Nausea ☐ Flatulence
☐ Vomiting
☐ Other ______________________

Stress Level

Sleep

Energy Level

Activity Level

Pain Location (If Applicable)

☐ Abdomen ☐ Joints
☐ Stomach ☐ Rectum
☐ Other ______________________

Medications

Notes

Daily Tracking

DATE:

S M T W T F S

Fluid Tracker 8 oz 8 oz 8 oz 8 oz 8 oz 8 oz 8 oz 8 oz

Meal Tracking

Time	Meal	Pain Scale 0-5 0= No pain 5= Severe
BREAKFAST		
LUNCH		
DINNER		
SNACKS		

Bowel Activity

Normal	Very Hard	Abnormalities
		☐ Blood ☐ Mucus ☐ Other ____
		☐ Blood ☐ Mucus ☐ Other ____
		☐ Blood ☐ Mucus ☐ Other ____
		☐ Blood ☐ Mucus ☐ Other ____
	More?	

Other Symptoms

☐ Bloating ☐ Fatigue
☐ Nausea ☐ Flatulence
☐ Vomiting
☐ Other ____________________

Stress Level

Sleep

Energy Level

Activity Level

Pain Location (If Applicable)

☐ Abdomen ☐ Joints
☐ Stomach ☐ Rectum
☐ Other ____________________

Notes

Medications

____
____
____
____
____

Daily Tracking

DATE:

S M T W T F S

Fluid Tracker 8 oz 8 oz 8 oz 8 oz 8 oz 8 oz 8 oz 8 oz

Meal Tracking

Time	Meal	Pain Scale 0-5 0= No pain 5= Severe
BREAKFAST		
LUNCH		
DINNER		
SNACKS		

Bowel Activity

Normal	Very Hard	Abnormalities
		☐ Blood ☐ Mucus ☐ Other ______
		☐ Blood ☐ Mucus ☐ Other ______
		☐ Blood ☐ Mucus ☐ Other ______
		☐ Blood ☐ Mucus ☐ Other ______
	More?	

Other Symptoms

☐ Bloating ☐ Fatigue
☐ Nausea ☐ Flatulence
☐ Vomiting
☐ Other ______________________

Pain Location (If Applicable)

☐ Abdomen ☐ Joints
☐ Stomach ☐ Rectum
☐ Other ______________________

Stress Level

Sleep

Energy Level

Activity Level

Medications

____
____
____
____
____

Notes

Daily Tracking

DATE:

S M T W T F S

Fluid Tracker 8 oz 8 oz 8 oz 8 oz 8 oz 8 oz 8 oz 8 oz

Meal Tracking

Time	Meal	Pain Scale 0-5 0= No pain 5= Severe
BREAKFAST		
LUNCH		
DINNER		
SNACKS		

Bowel Activity

Normal	Very Hard	Abnormalities
		☐ Blood ☐ Mucus ☐ Other ______
		☐ Blood ☐ Mucus ☐ Other ______
		☐ Blood ☐ Mucus ☐ Other ______
		☐ Blood ☐ Mucus ☐ Other ______
	More?	

Other Symptoms

☐ Bloating ☐ Fatigue
☐ Nausea ☐ Flatulence
☐ Vomiting
☐ Other ______________________

Stress Level

Sleep

Energy Level

Activity Level

Pain Location (If Applicable)

☐ Abdomen ☐ Joints
☐ Stomach ☐ Rectum
☐ Other ______________________

Medications

____
____
____
____
____

Notes

Daily Tracking

DATE:

S M T W T F S

Fluid Tracker: 8 oz | 8 oz | 8 oz | 8 oz | 8 oz | 8 oz | 8 oz | 8 oz

Meal Tracking

Time	Meal	Pain Scale 0-5 0= No pain 5= Severe
BREAKFAST		
LUNCH		
DINNER		
SNACKS		

Bowel Activity

Normal … Very Hard		Abnormalities
		☐ Blood ☐ Mucus ☐ Other ______
		☐ Blood ☐ Mucus ☐ Other ______
		☐ Blood ☐ Mucus ☐ Other ______
		☐ Blood ☐ Mucus ☐ Other ______
	More?	

Other Symptoms

- ☐ Bloating
- ☐ Fatigue
- ☐ Nausea
- ☐ Flatulence
- ☐ Vomiting
- ☐ Other ______________________

Stress Level

Sleep

Energy Level

Activity Level

Pain Location (If Applicable)

- ☐ Abdomen
- ☐ Joints
- ☐ Stomach
- ☐ Rectum
- ☐ Other ______________________

Medications

____

____

____

____

____

Notes

Daily Tracking

DATE:

S M T W T F S

Fluid Tracker 8 oz 8 oz 8 oz 8 oz 8 oz 8 oz 8 oz 8 oz

Meal Tracking

Time	Meal	Pain Scale 0-5 0= No pain 5= Severe
BREAKFAST		
LUNCH		
DINNER		
SNACKS		

Bowel Activity

Normal	Very Hard	Abnormalities
		☐ Blood ☐ Mucus ☐ Other ____
		☐ Blood ☐ Mucus ☐ Other ____
		☐ Blood ☐ Mucus ☐ Other ____
		☐ Blood ☐ Mucus ☐ Other ____
	More?	

Other Symptoms

☐ Bloating ☐ Fatigue
☐ Nausea ☐ Flatulence
☐ Vomiting
☐ Other ____________________

Stress Level

Sleep

Energy Level

Activity Level

Pain Location (If Applicable)

☐ Abdomen ☐ Joints
☐ Stomach ☐ Rectum
☐ Other ____________________

Medications

Notes

Daily Tracking

DATE:

S M T W T F S

Fluid Tracker: 8 oz | 8 oz | 8 oz | 8 oz | 8 oz | 8 oz | 8 oz | 8 oz

Meal Tracking

Time	Meal	Pain Scale 0-5 0= No pain 5= Severe
BREAKFAST		
LUNCH		
DINNER		
SNACKS		

Bowel Activity

Normal	Very Hard	Abnormalities
		☐ Blood ☐ Mucus ☐ Other ______
		☐ Blood ☐ Mucus ☐ Other ______
		☐ Blood ☐ Mucus ☐ Other ______
		☐ Blood ☐ Mucus ☐ Other ______
	More?	

Other Symptoms

- ☐ Bloating
- ☐ Fatigue
- ☐ Nausea
- ☐ Flatulence
- ☐ Vomiting
- ☐ Other ______________________

Stress Level

Sleep

Energy Level

Activity Level

Pain Location (If Applicable)

- ☐ Abdomen
- ☐ Joints
- ☐ Stomach
- ☐ Rectum
- ☐ Other ______________________

Medications

____

____

____

____

____

Notes

Weekly Reflections

What was the best thing that happened this week?

What was the hardest thing that happened this week?

What helped you the most this week?

What gave you hope this week?

What's one small win you can celebrate?

Was there something that eased your stress?

Overall, this week I felt

☐ A little better ☐ A lot better ☐ A little worse ☐ A lot worse
☐ About the same

Next week I want to:

____

____

____

____

Each note you write is a gift to your future self. You're building a record of wisdom.

Monthly Thoughts

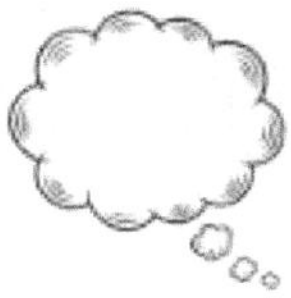

This page is your space to step back and see the bigger picture. Each month brings its own challenges and small victories—use this space to notice patterns, celebrate progress, and reflect on what your body and mind are teaching you. These notes can guide you forward with greater clarity and self-compassion.

This Month I Noticed...

(Write down patterns in your symptoms, energy, or mood.)

Biggest Challenge: ______________________________

____

Brightest Moment: ______________________________

____

Triggers I Noticed: ______________________________

____

Things That Helped: ______________________________

____

Medication / Treatment Notes: (Any changes, side effects, or adjustments.) ______________________________

____

____

Self-Care Check-In

How well I cared for myself this month: ______________________________

____

Looking Forward

Next month I want to focus on: ______________________________

____

____

Symptom Overview

Good Days: ________ Mild Days: ________ Flare Days: ________

Even in uncertainty, you are learning what your body needs.

Daily Tracking

DATE:

S M T W T F S

Fluid Tracker 8 oz 8 oz 8 oz 8 oz 8 oz 8 oz 8 oz 8 oz

Meal Tracking

Time	Meal	Pain Scale 0-5 0= No pain 5= Severe
BREAKFAST		
LUNCH		
DINNER		
SNACKS		

Bowel Activity

Normal	Very Hard	Abnormalities
		☐ Blood ☐ Mucus ☐ Other ________
		☐ Blood ☐ Mucus ☐ Other ________
		☐ Blood ☐ Mucus ☐ Other ________
		☐ Blood ☐ Mucus ☐ Other ________
	More?	

Other Symptoms

☐ Bloating ☐ Fatigue
☐ Nausea ☐ Flatulence
☐ Vomiting
☐ Other ____________________

Stress Level

Sleep

Energy Level

Activity Leve

Pain Location (If Applicable)

☐ Abdomen ☐ Joints
☐ Stomach ☐ Rectum
☐ Other ____________________

Medications

____
____
____
____
____

Notes

Daily Tracking

DATE:

S M T W T F S

Fluid Tracker: 8 oz | 8 oz | 8 oz | 8 oz | 8 oz | 8 oz | 8 oz | 8 oz

Meal Tracking

Time	Meal	Pain Scale 0-5 0= No pain 5= Severe
BREAKFAST		
LUNCH		
DINNER		
SNACKS		

Bowel Activity

Normal	Very Hard	Abnormalities
		☐ Blood ☐ Mucus ☐ Other ______
		☐ Blood ☐ Mucus ☐ Other ______
		☐ Blood ☐ Mucus ☐ Other ______
		☐ Blood ☐ Mucus ☐ Other ______
	More?	

Other Symptoms

☐ Bloating ☐ Fatigue
☐ Nausea ☐ Flatulence
☐ Vomiting
☐ Other ______________________

Stress Level

Sleep

Energy Level

Activity Level

Pain Location (If Applicable)

☐ Abdomen ☐ Joints
☐ Stomach ☐ Rectum
☐ Other ______________________

Medications

____
____
____
____
____

Notes

Daily Tracking

DATE:

S M T W T F S

Fluid Tracker: 8 oz | 8 oz | 8 oz | 8 oz | 8 oz | 8 oz | 8 oz | 8 oz

Meal Tracking

Time	Meal	Pain Scale 0-5 0= No pain 5= Severe
BREAKFAST		
LUNCH		
DINNER		
SNACKS		

Bowel Activity

Normal	Very Hard	Abnormalities
		☐ Blood ☐ Mucus ☐ Other ______
		☐ Blood ☐ Mucus ☐ Other ______
		☐ Blood ☐ Mucus ☐ Other ______
		☐ Blood ☐ Mucus ☐ Other ______
	More?	

Other Symptoms

- ☐ Bloating
- ☐ Fatigue
- ☐ Nausea
- ☐ Flatulence
- ☐ Vomiting
- ☐ Other ______________________

Stress Level

Sleep

Energy Level

Activity Level

Pain Location (If Applicable)

- ☐ Abdomen
- ☐ Joints
- ☐ Stomach
- ☐ Rectum
- ☐ Other ______________________

Notes

Medications

____

____

____

____

____

Daily Tracking

DATE: ______________________

S M T W T F S

Fluid Tracker 8 oz 8 oz 8 oz 8 oz 8 oz 8 oz 8 oz 8 oz

Meal Tracking

Time	Meal	Pain Scale 0-5 0= No pain 5= Severe
BREAKFAST		
LUNCH		
DINNER		
SNACKS		

Bowel Activity

Normal	Very Hard	Abnormalities
		☐ Blood ☐ Mucus ☐ Other ______
		☐ Blood ☐ Mucus ☐ Other ______
		☐ Blood ☐ Mucus ☐ Other ______
		☐ Blood ☐ Mucus ☐ Other ______
	More?	

Pain Location (If Applicable)

☐ Abdomen ☐ Joints
☐ Stomach ☐ Rectum
☐ Other ______________________

Notes

Other Symptoms

☐ Bloating ☐ Fatigue
☐ Nausea ☐ Flatulence
☐ Vomiting
☐ Other ______________________

Stress Level

Sleep

Energy Level

Activity Level

Medications

____
____
____
____
____

Daily Tracking

DATE:

S M T W T F S

Fluid Tracker 8 oz 8 oz 8 oz 8 oz 8 oz 8 oz 8 oz 8 oz

Meal Tracking

Time	Meal	Pain Scale 0-5 0= No pain 5= Severe
BREAKFAST		
LUNCH		
DINNER		
SNACKS		

Bowel Activity

Normal	Very Hard	Abnormalities
		☐ Blood ☐ Mucus ☐ Other
		☐ Blood ☐ Mucus ☐ Other
		☐ Blood ☐ Mucus ☐ Other
		☐ Blood ☐ Mucus ☐ Other
	More?	

Other Symptoms

☐ Bloating ☐ Fatigue
☐ Nausea ☐ Flatulence
☐ Vomiting
☐ Other ______

Stress Level

Sleep

Energy Level

Activity Leve

Pain Location (If Applicable)

☐ Abdomen ☐ Joints
☐ Stomach ☐ Rectum
☐ Other ______

Notes

Medications

Daily Tracking

DATE:

S M T W T F S

Fluid Tracker: 8 oz | 8 oz | 8 oz | 8 oz | 8 oz | 8 oz | 8 oz | 8 oz

Meal Tracking

Time	Meal	Pain Scale 0-5 0= No pain 5= Severe
BREAKFAST		
LUNCH		
DINNER		
SNACKS		

Bowel Activity

Normal	Very Hard	Abnormalities
		☐ Blood ☐ Mucus ☐ Other ____
		☐ Blood ☐ Mucus ☐ Other ____
		☐ Blood ☐ Mucus ☐ Other ____
		☐ Blood ☐ Mucus ☐ Other ____
	More?	

Other Symptoms

☐ Bloating ☐ Fatigue
☐ Nausea ☐ Flatulence
☐ Vomiting
☐ Other ____________________

Stress Level

Sleep

Energy Level

Activity Level

Pain Location (If Applicable)

☐ Abdomen ☐ Joints
☐ Stomach ☐ Rectum
☐ Other ____________________

Medications

____
____
____
____
____

Notes

Daily Tracking

DATE:

S M T W T F S

Fluid Tracker: 8 oz | 8 oz | 8 oz | 8 oz | 8 oz | 8 oz | 8 oz | 8 oz

Meal Tracking

Time	Meal	Pain Scale 0-5 0= No pain 5= Severe
BREAKFAST		
LUNCH		
DINNER		
SNACKS		

Bowel Activity

Normal	Very Hard	Abnormalities
		☐ Blood ☐ Mucus ☐ Other ______
		☐ Blood ☐ Mucus ☐ Other ______
		☐ Blood ☐ Mucus ☐ Other ______
		☐ Blood ☐ Mucus ☐ Other ______
	More?	

Other Symptoms

- ☐ Bloating
- ☐ Fatigue
- ☐ Nausea
- ☐ Flatulence
- ☐ Vomiting
- ☐ Other ______

Stress Level

Sleep

Energy Level

Activity Level

Pain Location (If Applicable)

- ☐ Abdomen
- ☐ Joints
- ☐ Stomach
- ☐ Rectum
- ☐ Other ______

Medications

______

______

______

______

______

Notes

Weekly Reflections

What was the best thing that happened this week?

What was the hardest thing that happened this week?

What helped you the most this week?

What gave you hope this week?

What's one small win you can celebrate?

Was there something that eased your stress?

Overall, this week I felt

- ☐ A little better
- ☐ A lot better
- ☐ A little worse
- ☐ A lot worse
- ☐ About the same

Next week I want to:

____

____

____

____

Even storms pass. Trust that better moments are ahead.

Daily Tracking

DATE:

S M T W T F S

Fluid Tracker 8 oz 8 oz 8 oz 8 oz 8 oz 8 oz 8 oz 8 oz

Meal Tracking

Time	Meal	Pain Scale 0-5 0= No pain 5= Severe
BREAKFAST		
LUNCH		
DINNER		
SNACKS		

Bowel Activity

Normal	Very Hard	Abnormalities
		☐ Blood ☐ Mucus ☐ Other ______
		☐ Blood ☐ Mucus ☐ Other ______
		☐ Blood ☐ Mucus ☐ Other ______
		☐ Blood ☐ Mucus ☐ Other ______
	More?	

Other Symptoms

☐ Bloating ☐ Fatigue
☐ Nausea ☐ Flatulence
☐ Vomiting
☐ Other ______________________

Stress Level

Sleep

Energy Level

Activity Level

Pain Location (If Applicable)

☐ Abdomen ☐ Joints
☐ Stomach ☐ Rectum
☐ Other ______________________

Medications

____

____

____

____

____

Notes

Daily Tracking

DATE:

S M T W T F S

Fluid Tracker: 8 oz | 8 oz | 8 oz | 8 oz | 8 oz | 8 oz | 8 oz | 8 oz

Meal Tracking

Time	Meal	Pain Scale 0-5 0= No pain 5= Severe
BREAKFAST		
LUNCH		
DINNER		
SNACKS		

Bowel Activity

Normal	Very Hard	Abnormalities
		☐ Blood ☐ Mucus ☐ Other ______
		☐ Blood ☐ Mucus ☐ Other ______
		☐ Blood ☐ Mucus ☐ Other ______
		☐ Blood ☐ Mucus ☐ Other ______
	More?	

Other Symptoms

☐ Bloating ☐ Fatigue
☐ Nausea ☐ Flatulence
☐ Vomiting
☐ Other ______________________

Stress Level

Sleep

Energy Level

Activity Level

Pain Location (If Applicable)

☐ Abdomen ☐ Joints
☐ Stomach ☐ Rectum
☐ Other ______________________

Medications

____
____
____
____
____

Notes

Daily Tracking

DATE:

S M T W T F S

Fluid Tracker 8 oz 8 oz 8 oz 8 oz 8 oz 8 oz 8 oz 8 oz

Meal Tracking

Time	Meal	Pain Scale 0-5 0= No pain 5= Severe
BREAKFAST		
LUNCH		
DINNER		
SNACKS		

Bowel Activity

Normal	Very Hard	Abnormalities
		☐ Blood ☐ Mucus ☐ Other
		☐ Blood ☐ Mucus ☐ Other
		☐ Blood ☐ Mucus ☐ Other
		☐ Blood ☐ Mucus ☐ Other
	More?	

Pain Location (If Applicable)

☐ Abdomen ☐ Joints
☐ Stomach ☐ Rectum
☐ Other ______

Notes

Other Symptoms

☐ Bloating ☐ Fatigue
☐ Nausea ☐ Flatulence
☐ Vomiting
☐ Other ______

Stress Level

Sleep

Energy Level

Activity Level

Medications

______
______
______
______
______

Daily Tracking

DATE:

S M T W T F S

Fluid Tracker 8 oz 8 oz 8 oz 8 oz 8 oz 8 oz 8 oz 8 oz

Meal Tracking

Time	Meal	Pain Scale 0-5 0= No pain 5= Severe
BREAKFAST		
LUNCH		
DINNER		
SNACKS		

Bowel Activity

Normal	Very Hard	Abnormalities
		☐ Blood ☐ Mucus ☐ Other ______
		☐ Blood ☐ Mucus ☐ Other ______
		☐ Blood ☐ Mucus ☐ Other ______
		☐ Blood ☐ Mucus ☐ Other ______
	More?	

Other Symptoms

☐ Bloating ☐ Fatigue
☐ Nausea ☐ Flatulence
☐ Vomiting
☐ Other ______________________

Stress Level

Sleep

Energy Level

Activity Level

Pain Location (If Applicable)

☐ Abdomen ☐ Joints
☐ Stomach ☐ Rectum
☐ Other ______________________

Medications

____
____
____
____
____

Notes

Daily Tracking

DATE:

S M T W T F S

Fluid Tracker: 8 oz | 8 oz | 8 oz | 8 oz | 8 oz | 8 oz | 8 oz | 8 oz

Meal Tracking

Time	Meal	Pain Scale 0-5 0= No pain 5= Severe
BREAKFAST		
LUNCH		
DINNER		
SNACKS		

Bowel Activity

Normal	Very Hard	Abnormalities
		☐ Blood ☐ Mucus ☐ Other ______
		☐ Blood ☐ Mucus ☐ Other ______
		☐ Blood ☐ Mucus ☐ Other ______
		☐ Blood ☐ Mucus ☐ Other ______
	More?	

Other Symptoms

☐ Bloating ☐ Fatigue
☐ Nausea ☐ Flatulence
☐ Vomiting
☐ Other ______________________

Stress Level

Sleep

Energy Level

Activity Level

Pain Location (If Applicable)

☐ Abdomen ☐ Joints
☐ Stomach ☐ Rectum
☐ Other ______________________

Medications

____
____
____
____
____

Notes

Daily Tracking

DATE:

S M T W T F S

Fluid Tracker: 8 oz | 8 oz | 8 oz | 8 oz | 8 oz | 8 oz | 8 oz | 8 oz

Meal Tracking

Time	Meal	Pain Scale 0-5 0= No pain 5= Severe
BREAKFAST		
LUNCH		
DINNER		
SNACKS		

Bowel Activity

Normal	Very Hard	Abnormalities
		☐ Blood ☐ Mucus ☐ Other ______
		☐ Blood ☐ Mucus ☐ Other ______
		☐ Blood ☐ Mucus ☐ Other ______
		☐ Blood ☐ Mucus ☐ Other ______
	More?	

Other Symptoms

☐ Bloating ☐ Fatigue
☐ Nausea ☐ Flatulence
☐ Vomiting
☐ Other ______________________

Stress Level

Sleep

Energy Level

Activity Level

Pain Location (If Applicable)

☐ Abdomen ☐ Joints
☐ Stomach ☐ Rectum
☐ Other ______________________

Medications

____
____
____
____
____

Notes

Daily Tracking

DATE:

S M T W T F S

Fluid Tracker: 8 oz | 8 oz | 8 oz | 8 oz | 8 oz | 8 oz | 8 oz | 8 oz

Meal Tracking

Time	Meal	Pain Scale 0-5 0= No pain 5= Severe
BREAKFAST		
LUNCH		
DINNER		
SNACKS		

Bowel Activity

Normal	Very Hard	Abnormalities
		☐ Blood ☐ Mucus ☐ Other ______
		☐ Blood ☐ Mucus ☐ Other ______
		☐ Blood ☐ Mucus ☐ Other ______
		☐ Blood ☐ Mucus ☐ Other ______
	More?	

Other Symptoms

☐ Bloating ☐ Fatigue
☐ Nausea ☐ Flatulence
☐ Vomiting
☐ Other ______________________

Stress Level

Sleep

Energy Level

Activity Level

Pain Location (If Applicable)

☐ Abdomen ☐ Joints
☐ Stomach ☐ Rectum
☐ Other ______________________

Medications

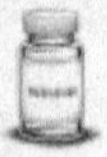

____
____
____
____
____

Notes

Weekly Reflections

What was the best thing that happened this week?

What was the hardest thing that happened this week?

What helped you the most this week?

What gave you hope this week?

What's one small win you can celebrate?

Was there something that eased your stress?

Overall, this week I felt

☐ A little better ☐ A lot better ☐ A little worse ☐ A lot worse
☐ About the same

Next week I want to:

Self-compassion is as important as any routine. Be as kind to yourself as you would to a friend.

Daily Tracking

DATE:

S M T W T F S

Fluid Tracker: 8 oz | 8 oz | 8 oz | 8 oz | 8 oz | 8 oz | 8 oz | 8 oz

Meal Tracking

Time	Meal	Pain Scale 0-5 0= No pain 5= Severe
BREAKFAST		
LUNCH		
DINNER		
SNACKS		

Bowel Activity

Normal	Very Hard	Abnormalities
		☐ Blood ☐ Mucus ☐ Other ______
		☐ Blood ☐ Mucus ☐ Other ______
		☐ Blood ☐ Mucus ☐ Other ______
		☐ Blood ☐ Mucus ☐ Other ______
	More?	

Other Symptoms

☐ Bloating ☐ Fatigue
☐ Nausea ☐ Flatulence
☐ Vomiting
☐ Other ______________________

Stress Level

Sleep

Energy Level

Activity Leve

Pain Location (If Applicable)

☐ Abdomen ☐ Joints
☐ Stomach ☐ Rectum
☐ Other ______________________

Medications

____
____
____
____
____

Notes

Daily Tracking

DATE:

S M T W T F S

Fluid Tracker: 8 oz | 8 oz | 8 oz | 8 oz | 8 oz | 8 oz | 8 oz | 8 oz

Meal Tracking

Time	Meal	Pain Scale 0-5 0= No pain 5= Severe
BREAKFAST		
LUNCH		
DINNER		
SNACKS		

Bowel Activity

Normal	Very Hard	Abnormalities
		☐ Blood ☐ Mucus ☐ Other ______
		☐ Blood ☐ Mucus ☐ Other ______
		☐ Blood ☐ Mucus ☐ Other ______
		☐ Blood ☐ Mucus ☐ Other ______
	More?	

Pain Location (If Applicable)

- ☐ Abdomen
- ☐ Joints
- ☐ Stomach
- ☐ Rectum
- ☐ Other ______________________

Notes

Other Symptoms

- ☐ Bloating
- ☐ Fatigue
- ☐ Nausea
- ☐ Flatulence
- ☐ Vomiting
- ☐ Other ______________________

Stress Level

Sleep

Energy Level

Activity Level

Medications

____

____

____

____

____

Daily Tracking

DATE:

S M T W T F S

Fluid Tracker 8 oz 8 oz 8 oz 8 oz 8 oz 8 oz 8 oz 8 oz

Meal Tracking

Time	Meal	Pain Scale 0-5 0= No pain 5= Severe
BREAKFAST		
LUNCH		
DINNER		
SNACKS		

Bowel Activity

Normal	Very Hard	Abnormalities
		Blood Mucus Other
		Blood Mucus Other
		Blood Mucus Other
		Blood Mucus Other
	More?	

Other Symptoms

- ☐ Bloating
- ☐ Fatigue
- ☐ Nausea
- ☐ Flatulence
- ☐ Vomiting
- ☐ Other ______

Stress Level

Sleep

Energy Level

Activity Level

Pain Location (If Applicable)

- ☐ Abdomen
- ☐ Joints
- ☐ Stomach
- ☐ Rectum
- ☐ Other ______

Medications

Notes

Daily Tracking

DATE:

S M T W T F S

Fluid Tracker 8 oz 8 oz 8 oz 8 oz 8 oz 8 oz 8 oz 8 oz

Meal Tracking

Time	Meal	Pain Scale 0-5 0= No pain 5= Severe
BREAKFAST		
LUNCH		
DINNER		
SNACKS		

Bowel Activity

Normal	Very Hard	Abnormalities
		☐ Blood ☐ Mucus ☐ Other ______
		☐ Blood ☐ Mucus ☐ Other ______
		☐ Blood ☐ Mucus ☐ Other ______
		☐ Blood ☐ Mucus ☐ Other ______
	More?	

Other Symptoms

☐ Bloating ☐ Fatigue
☐ Nausea ☐ Flatulence
☐ Vomiting
☐ Other ______________________

Stress Level

Sleep

Energy Level

Activity Level

Pain Location (If Applicable)

☐ Abdomen ☐ Joints
☐ Stomach ☐ Rectum
☐ Other ______________________

Medications

____
____
____
____
____

Notes

Daily Tracking

DATE:

S M T W T F S

Fluid Tracker 8 oz 8 oz 8 oz 8 oz 8 oz 8 oz 8 oz 8 oz

Meal Tracking

Time	Meal	Pain Scale 0-5 0= No pain 5= Severe
BREAKFAST		
LUNCH		
DINNER		
SNACKS		

Bowel Activity

Normal	Very Hard	Abnormalities
		☐ Blood ☐ Mucus ☐ Other ______
		☐ Blood ☐ Mucus ☐ Other ______
		☐ Blood ☐ Mucus ☐ Other ______
		☐ Blood ☐ Mucus ☐ Other ______
	More?	

Other Symptoms

☐ Bloating ☐ Fatigue
☐ Nausea ☐ Flatulence
☐ Vomiting
☐ Other ______________________

Stress Level

Sleep

Energy Level

Activity Level

Pain Location (If Applicable)

☐ Abdomen ☐ Joints
☐ Stomach ☐ Rectum
☐ Other ______________________

Medications

Notes

Daily Tracking

DATE:

S M T W T F S

Meal Tracking

Fluid Tracker: 8 oz | 8 oz | 8 oz | 8 oz | 8 oz | 8 oz | 8 oz | 8 oz

Time	Meal	Pain Scale 0-5 0= No pain 5= Severe
BREAKFAST		
LUNCH		
DINNER		
SNACKS		

Bowel Activity

Normal	Very Hard	Abnormalities
		☐ Blood ☐ Mucus ☐ Other ____
		☐ Blood ☐ Mucus ☐ Other ____
		☐ Blood ☐ Mucus ☐ Other ____
		☐ Blood ☐ Mucus ☐ Other ____
	More?	

Other Symptoms

- ☐ Bloating
- ☐ Fatigue
- ☐ Nausea
- ☐ Flatulence
- ☐ Vomiting
- ☐ Other ____________________

Stress Level

Sleep

Energy Level

Activity Level

Pain Location (If Applicable)

- ☐ Abdomen
- ☐ Joints
- ☐ Stomach
- ☐ Rectum
- ☐ Other ____________________

Notes

Medications

____

____

____

____

____

Daily Tracking

DATE:

S M T W T F S

Fluid Tracker 8 oz 8 oz 8 oz 8 oz 8 oz 8 oz 8 oz 8 oz

Meal Tracking

Time	Meal	Pain Scale 0-5 0= No pain 5= Severe
BREAKFAST		
LUNCH		
DINNER		
SNACKS		

Bowel Activity

Normal	Very Hard	Abnormalities
		☐ Blood ☐ Mucus ☐ Other ____
		☐ Blood ☐ Mucus ☐ Other ____
		☐ Blood ☐ Mucus ☐ Other ____
		☐ Blood ☐ Mucus ☐ Other ____
	More?	

Other Symptoms

☐ Bloating ☐ Fatigue
☐ Nausea ☐ Flatulence
☐ Vomiting
☐ Other ____

Stress Level

Sleep

Energy Level

Activity Level

Pain Location (If Applicable)

☐ Abdomen ☐ Joints
☐ Stomach ☐ Rectum
☐ Other ____

Medications

____
____
____
____
____

Notes

Weekly Reflections

What was the best thing that happened this week?

What was the hardest thing that happened this week?

What helped you the most this week?

What gave you hope this week?

What's one small win you can celebrate?

Was there something that eased your stress?

Overall, this week I felt

☐ A little better ☐ A lot better ☐ A little worse ☐ A lot worse

☐ About the same

Next week I want to:

____

____

____

____

What you're carrying is real, and so is your strength. Take pride in both.

Daily Tracking

DATE:

S M T W T F S

Fluid Tracker 8 oz 8 oz 8 oz 8 oz 8 oz 8 oz 8 oz 8 oz

Meal Tracking

Time	Meal	Pain Scale 0-5 0= No pain 5= Severe
BREAKFAST		
LUNCH		
DINNER		
SNACKS		

Bowel Activity

Normal	Very Hard	Abnormalities
		☐ Blood ☐ Mucus ☐ Other ______
		☐ Blood ☐ Mucus ☐ Other ______
		☐ Blood ☐ Mucus ☐ Other ______
		☐ Blood ☐ Mucus ☐ Other ______
	More?	

Other Symptoms

☐ Bloating ☐ Fatigue
☐ Nausea ☐ Flatulence
☐ Vomiting
☐ Other ______________________

Stress Level

Sleep

Energy Level

Activity Level

Pain Location (If Applicable)

☐ Abdomen ☐ Joints
☐ Stomach ☐ Rectum
☐ Other ______________________

Medications

____
____
____
____
____

Notes

Daily Tracking

DATE:

S M T W T F S

Fluid Tracker: 8 oz | 8 oz | 8 oz | 8 oz | 8 oz | 8 oz | 8 oz | 8 oz

Meal Tracking

Time	Meal	Pain Scale 0-5 0= No pain 5= Severe
BREAKFAST		
LUNCH		
DINNER		
SNACKS		

Bowel Activity

Normal	Very Hard	Abnormalities
		☐ Blood ☐ Mucus ☐ Other ______
		☐ Blood ☐ Mucus ☐ Other ______
		☐ Blood ☐ Mucus ☐ Other ______
		☐ Blood ☐ Mucus ☐ Other ______
	More?	

Other Symptoms

☐ Bloating ☐ Fatigue
☐ Nausea ☐ Flatulence
☐ Vomiting
☐ Other ________________

Stress Level

Sleep

Energy Level

Activity Level

Pain Location (If Applicable)

☐ Abdomen ☐ Joints
☐ Stomach ☐ Rectum
☐ Other ________________

Medications

Notes

Daily Tracking

DATE:

S M T W T F S

Fluid Tracker: 8 oz | 8 oz | 8 oz | 8 oz | 8 oz | 8 oz | 8 oz | 8 oz

Meal Tracking

Time	Meal	Pain Scale 0-5 0= No pain 5= Severe
BREAKFAST		
LUNCH		
DINNER		
SNACKS		

Bowel Activity

Normal	Very Hard	Abnormalities
		☐ Blood ☐ Mucus ☐ Other
		☐ Blood ☐ Mucus ☐ Other
		☐ Blood ☐ Mucus ☐ Other
		☐ Blood ☐ Mucus ☐ Other
	More?	

Other Symptoms

☐ Bloating ☐ Fatigue
☐ Nausea ☐ Flatulence
☐ Vomiting
☐ Other ______

Stress Level

Sleep

Energy Level

Activity Level

Pain Location (If Applicable)

☐ Abdomen ☐ Joints
☐ Stomach ☐ Rectum
☐ Other ______

Medications

Notes

Daily Tracking

DATE:

S M T W T F S

Meal Tracking

Fluid Tracker 8 oz 8 oz 8 oz 8 oz 8 oz 8 oz 8 oz 8 oz

Time	Meal	Pain Scale 0-5 0= No pain 5= Severe
BREAKFAST		
LUNCH		
DINNER		
SNACKS		

Bowel Activity

Normal	Very Hard	Abnormalities
		◻ Blood ◻ Mucus ◻ Other ______
		◻ Blood ◻ Mucus ◻ Other ______
		◻ Blood ◻ Mucus ◻ Other ______
		◻ Blood ◻ Mucus ◻ Other ______
	More?	

Other Symptoms

☐ Bloating ☐ Fatigue
☐ Nausea ☐ Flatulence
☐ Vomiting
☐ Other ______________________

Stress Level

Sleep

Energy Level

Activity Level

Pain Location (If Applicable)

☐ Abdomen ☐ Joints
☐ Stomach ☐ Rectum
☐ Other ______________________

Medications

____
____
____
____
____

Notes

Daily Tracking

DATE:

S M T W T F S

Fluid Tracker 8 oz 8 oz 8 oz 8 oz 8 oz 8 oz 8 oz 8 oz

Meal Tracking

Time	Meal	Pain Scale 0-5 0= No pain 5= Severe
BREAKFAST		
LUNCH		
DINNER		
SNACKS		

Bowel Activity

Normal	Very Hard	Abnormalities
		☐ Blood ☐ Mucus ☐ Other ______
		☐ Blood ☐ Mucus ☐ Other ______
		☐ Blood ☐ Mucus ☐ Other ______
		☐ Blood ☐ Mucus ☐ Other ______
	More?	

Other Symptoms

☐ Bloating ☐ Fatigue
☐ Nausea ☐ Flatulence
☐ Vomiting
☐ Other ______________________

Stress Level

Sleep

Energy Level

Activity Level

Pain Location (If Applicable)

☐ Abdomen ☐ Joints
☐ Stomach ☐ Rectum
☐ Other ______________________

Medications

Notes

Daily Tracking

DATE:

(S) (M) (T) (W) (T) (F) (S)

Fluid Tracker: 8 oz | 8 oz | 8 oz | 8 oz | 8 oz | 8 oz | 8 oz | 8 oz

Meal Tracking

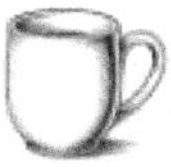

Time	Meal	Pain Scale 0-5 0= No pain 5= Severe
BREAKFAST		
LUNCH		
DINNER		
SNACKS		

Bowel Activity

Normal	Very Hard	Abnormalities
		☐ Blood ☐ Mucus ☐ Other ______
		☐ Blood ☐ Mucus ☐ Other ______
		☐ Blood ☐ Mucus ☐ Other ______
		☐ Blood ☐ Mucus ☐ Other ______
	More?	

Other Symptoms

☐ Bloating ☐ Fatigue
☐ Nausea ☐ Flatulence
☐ Vomiting
☐ Other ______________________

Stress Level

Sleep

Energy Level

Activity Level

Pain Location (If Applicable)

☐ Abdomen ☐ Joints
☐ Stomach ☐ Rectum
☐ Other ______________________

Medications

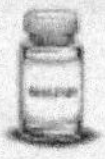

____
____
____
____
____

Notes

Daily Tracking

DATE:

S M T W T F S

Fluid Tracker 8 oz 8 oz 8 oz 8 oz 8 oz 8 oz 8 oz 8 oz

Meal Tracking

Time	Meal	Pain Scale 0-5 0= No pain 5= Severe
BREAKFAST		
LUNCH		
DINNER		
SNACKS		

Bowel Activity

Normal	Very Hard	Abnormalities
		☐ Blood ☐ Mucus ☐ Other ______
		☐ Blood ☐ Mucus ☐ Other ______
		☐ Blood ☐ Mucus ☐ Other ______
		☐ Blood ☐ Mucus ☐ Other ______
	More?	

Other Symptoms

☐ Bloating ☐ Fatigue
☐ Nausea ☐ Flatulence
☐ Vomiting
☐ Other ______

Stress Level

Sleep

Energy Level

Activity Level

Pain Location (If Applicable)

☐ Abdomen ☐ Joints
☐ Stomach ☐ Rectum
☐ Other ______

Medications

______
______
______
______
______

Notes

Weekly Reflections

What was the best thing that happened this week?

What was the hardest thing that happened this week?

What helped you the most this week?

What gave you hope this week?

What's one small win you can celebrate?

Was there something that eased your stress?

Overall, this week I felt

☐ A little better ☐ A lot better ☐ A little worse ☐ A lot worse
☐ About the same

Next week I want to:

____

____

____

____

A journal is more than paper—it's a place where your courage takes shape.

Monthly Thoughts

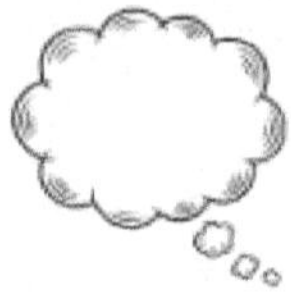

This page is your space to step back and see the bigger picture. Each month brings its own challenges and small victories—use this space to notice patterns, celebrate progress, and reflect on what your body and mind are teaching you. These notes can guide you forward with greater clarity and self-compassion.

This Month I Noticed...

(Write down patterns in your symptoms, energy, or mood.)

Biggest Challenge: ____

____

Brightest Moment: ____

____

Triggers I Noticed: ____

____

Things That Helped: ____

____

Medication / Treatment Notes: (Any changes, side effects, or adjustments.) ____

____

____

Self-Care Check-In

How well I cared for myself this month: ____________________

____

Looking Forward

Next month I want to focus on: ____________________________

____

____

Symptom Overview

Good Days: ________ Mild Days: ________ Flare Days: ________

The slowest growth is often the strongest.

Daily Tracking

DATE:

S M T W T F S

Fluid Tracker 8 oz 8 oz 8 oz 8 oz 8 oz 8 oz 8 oz 8 oz

Meal Tracking

Time	Meal	Pain Scale 0-5 0= No pain 5= Severe
BREAKFAST		
LUNCH		
DINNER		
SNACKS		

Bowel Activity

Normal	Very Hard	Abnormalities
		☐ Blood ☐ Mucus ☐ Other ______
		☐ Blood ☐ Mucus ☐ Other ______
		☐ Blood ☐ Mucus ☐ Other ______
		☐ Blood ☐ Mucus ☐ Other ______
	More?	

Other Symptoms

☐ Bloating ☐ Fatigue
☐ Nausea ☐ Flatulence
☐ Vomiting
☐ Other ______________________

Stress Level

Sleep

Energy Level

Activity Level

Pain Location (If Applicable)

☐ Abdomen ☐ Joints
☐ Stomach ☐ Rectum
☐ Other ______________________

Medications

____
____
____
____
____

Notes

Daily Tracking

DATE:

S M T W T F S

Fluid Tracker 8 oz 8 oz 8 oz 8 oz 8 oz 8 oz 8 oz 8 oz

Meal Tracking

Time	Meal	Pain Scale 0-5 0= No pain 5= Severe
BREAKFAST		
LUNCH		
DINNER		
SNACKS		

Bowel Activity

Normal	Very Hard	Abnormalities
		☐ Blood ☐ Mucus ☐ Other ______
		☐ Blood ☐ Mucus ☐ Other ______
		☐ Blood ☐ Mucus ☐ Other ______
		☐ Blood ☐ Mucus ☐ Other ______
	More?	

Other Symptoms

☐ Bloating ☐ Fatigue
☐ Nausea ☐ Flatulence
☐ Vomiting
☐ Other ______________________

Stress Level

Sleep

Energy Level

Activity Level

Pain Location (If Applicable)

☐ Abdomen ☐ Joints
☐ Stomach ☐ Rectum
☐ Other ______________________

Medications

____
____
____
____
____

Notes

Daily Tracking

DATE:

S M T W T F S

Fluid Tracker 8 oz 8 oz 8 oz 8 oz 8 oz 8 oz 8 oz 8 oz

Meal Tracking

Time	Meal	Pain Scale 0-5 0= No pain 5= Severe
BREAKFAST		
LUNCH		
DINNER		
SNACKS		

Bowel Activity

Normal	Very Hard	Abnormalities
		☐ Blood ☐ Mucus ☐ Other ______
		☐ Blood ☐ Mucus ☐ Other ______
		☐ Blood ☐ Mucus ☐ Other ______
		☐ Blood ☐ Mucus ☐ Other ______
	More?	

Pain Location (If Applicable)

☐ Abdomen ☐ Joints
☐ Stomach ☐ Rectum
☐ Other ______________________

Notes

Other Symptoms

☐ Bloating ☐ Fatigue
☐ Nausea ☐ Flatulence
☐ Vomiting
☐ Other ______________________

Stress Level

Sleep

Energy Level

Activity Level

Medications

____
____
____
____
____

Daily Tracking

DATE:

S M T W T F S

Fluid Tracker 8 oz 8 oz 8 oz 8 oz 8 oz 8 oz 8 oz 8 oz

Meal Tracking

Time	Meal	Pain Scale 0-5 0= No pain 5= Severe
BREAKFAST		
LUNCH		
DINNER		
SNACKS		

Bowel Activity

Normal	Very Hard	Abnormalities
		☐ Blood ☐ Mucus ☐ Other ______
		☐ Blood ☐ Mucus ☐ Other ______
		☐ Blood ☐ Mucus ☐ Other ______
		☐ Blood ☐ Mucus ☐ Other ______
	More?	

Other Symptoms

☐ Bloating ☐ Fatigue
☐ Nausea ☐ Flatulence
☐ Vomiting
☐ Other ______

Stress Level

Sleep

Energy Level

Activity Leve

Pain Location (If Applicable)

☐ Abdomen ☐ Joints
☐ Stomach ☐ Rectum
☐ Other ______

Medications

______
______
______
______
______

Notes

Daily Tracking

DATE:

S M T W T F S

Fluid Tracker 8 oz 8 oz 8 oz 8 oz 8 oz 8 oz 8 oz 8 oz

Meal Tracking

Time	Meal	Pain Scale 0-5 0= No pain 5= Severe
BREAKFAST		
LUNCH		
DINNER		
SNACKS		

Bowel Activity

Normal	Very Hard	Abnormalities
		☐ Blood ☐ Mucus ☐ Other ______
		☐ Blood ☐ Mucus ☐ Other ______
		☐ Blood ☐ Mucus ☐ Other ______
		☐ Blood ☐ Mucus ☐ Other ______
	More?	

Other Symptoms

☐ Bloating ☐ Fatigue
☐ Nausea ☐ Flatulence
☐ Vomiting
☐ Other ______________________

Stress Level

Sleep

Energy Level

Activity Level

Pain Location (If Applicable)

☐ Abdomen ☐ Joints
☐ Stomach ☐ Rectum
☐ Other ______________________

Medications

____
____
____
____
____

Notes

Daily Tracking

DATE:

S M T W T F S

Fluid Tracker: 8 oz | 8 oz | 8 oz | 8 oz | 8 oz | 8 oz | 8 oz | 8 oz

Meal Tracking

Time	Meal	Pain Scale 0-5 0= No pain 5= Severe
BREAKFAST		
LUNCH		
DINNER		
SNACKS		

Bowel Activity

Normal	Very Hard	Abnormalities
		☐ Blood ☐ Mucus ☐ Other
		☐ Blood ☐ Mucus ☐ Other
		☐ Blood ☐ Mucus ☐ Other
		☐ Blood ☐ Mucus ☐ Other
	More?	

Other Symptoms

☐ Bloating ☐ Fatigue
☐ Nausea ☐ Flatulence
☐ Vomiting
☐ Other ______

Stress Level

Sleep

Energy Level

Activity Level

Pain Location (If Applicable)

☐ Abdomen ☐ Joints
☐ Stomach ☐ Rectum
☐ Other ______

Medications

______
______
______
______
______

Notes

Daily Tracking

DATE:

S M T W T F S

Fluid Tracker: 8 oz | 8 oz | 8 oz | 8 oz | 8 oz | 8 oz | 8 oz | 8 oz

Meal Tracking

Time	Meal	Pain Scale 0-5 0= No pain 5= Severe
BREAKFAST		
LUNCH		
DINNER		
SNACKS		

Bowel Activity

Normal	Very Hard	Abnormalities
		☐ Blood ☐ Mucus ☐ Other ______
		☐ Blood ☐ Mucus ☐ Other ______
		☐ Blood ☐ Mucus ☐ Other ______
		☐ Blood ☐ Mucus ☐ Other ______
	More?	

Other Symptoms

☐ Bloating ☐ Fatigue
☐ Nausea ☐ Flatulence
☐ Vomiting
☐ Other ______________________

Stress Level

Sleep

Energy Level

Activity Level

Pain Location (If Applicable)

☐ Abdomen ☐ Joints
☐ Stomach ☐ Rectum
☐ Other ______________________

Medications

____
____
____
____
____

Notes

Weekly Reflections

What was the best thing that happened this week?

What was the hardest thing that happened this week?

What helped you the most this week?

What gave you hope this week?

What's one small win you can celebrate?

Was there something that eased your stress?

Overall, this week I felt

☐ A little better ☐ A lot better ☐ A little worse ☐ A lot worse
☐ About the same

Next week I want to:

____

____

____

____

A journal is more than paper—it's a place where your courage takes shape.

Daily Tracking

DATE:

S M T W T F S

Meal Tracking

Fluid Tracker: 8 oz | 8 oz | 8 oz | 8 oz | 8 oz | 8 oz | 8 oz | 8 oz

Time	Meal	Pain Scale 0-5 0= No pain 5= Severe
BREAKFAST		
LUNCH		
DINNER		
SNACKS		

Bowel Activity

Normal	Very Hard	Abnormalities
		☐ Blood ☐ Mucus ☐ Other ______
		☐ Blood ☐ Mucus ☐ Other ______
		☐ Blood ☐ Mucus ☐ Other ______
		☐ Blood ☐ Mucus ☐ Other ______
	More?	

Other Symptoms

☐ Bloating ☐ Fatigue
☐ Nausea ☐ Flatulence
☐ Vomiting
☐ Other ______________________

Stress Level

Sleep

Energy Level

Activity Level

Pain Location (If Applicable)

☐ Abdomen ☐ Joints
☐ Stomach ☐ Rectum
☐ Other ______________________

Medications

____
____
____
____
____

Notes

Daily Tracking

DATE:

S M T W T F S

Fluid Tracker 8 oz 8 oz 8 oz 8 oz 8 oz 8 oz 8 oz 8 oz

Meal Tracking

Time	Meal	Pain Scale 0-5 0= No pain 5= Severe
BREAKFAST		
LUNCH		
DINNER		
SNACKS		

Bowel Activity

Normal	Very Hard	Abnormalities
		☐ Blood ☐ Mucus ☐ Other ______
		☐ Blood ☐ Mucus ☐ Other ______
		☐ Blood ☐ Mucus ☐ Other ______
		☐ Blood ☐ Mucus ☐ Other ______
	More?	

Other Symptoms

☐ Bloating ☐ Fatigue
☐ Nausea ☐ Flatulence
☐ Vomiting
☐ Other ______

Stress Level

Sleep

Energy Level

Activity Level

Pain Location (If Applicable)

☐ Abdomen ☐ Joints
☐ Stomach ☐ Rectum
☐ Other ______

Medications

______
______
______
______
______

Notes

Daily Tracking

DATE:

S M T W T F S

Fluid Tracker 8 oz 8 oz 8 oz 8 oz 8 oz 8 oz 8 oz 8 oz

Meal Tracking

Time	Meal	Pain Scale 0-5 0= No pain 5= Severe
BREAKFAST		
LUNCH		
DINNER		
SNACKS		

Bowel Activity

Normal	Very Hard	Abnormalities
		☐ Blood ☐ Mucus ☐ Other
		☐ Blood ☐ Mucus ☐ Other
		☐ Blood ☐ Mucus ☐ Other
		☐ Blood ☐ Mucus ☐ Other
	More?	

Other Symptoms

☐ Bloating ☐ Fatigue
☐ Nausea ☐ Flatulence
☐ Vomiting
☐ Other ____________________

Stress Level

Sleep

Energy Level

Activity Level

Pain Location (If Applicable)

☐ Abdomen ☐ Joints
☐ Stomach ☐ Rectum
☐ Other ____________________

Notes

Medications

____
____
____
____
____

Daily Tracking

DATE:

S M T W T F S

Fluid Tracker 8 oz 8 oz 8 oz 8 oz 8 oz 8 oz 8 oz 8 oz

Meal Tracking

Time	Meal	Pain Scale 0-5 0= No pain 5= Severe
BREAKFAST		
LUNCH		
DINNER		
SNACKS		

Bowel Activity

Normal	Very Hard	Abnormalities
		☐ Blood ☐ Mucus ☐ Other ______
		☐ Blood ☐ Mucus ☐ Other ______
		☐ Blood ☐ Mucus ☐ Other ______
		☐ Blood ☐ Mucus ☐ Other ______
	More?	

Other Symptoms

☐ Bloating ☐ Fatigue
☐ Nausea ☐ Flatulence
☐ Vomiting
☐ Other ______________________

Stress Level

Sleep

Energy Level

Activity Level

Pain Location (If Applicable)

☐ Abdomen ☐ Joints
☐ Stomach ☐ Rectum
☐ Other ______________________

Medications

____
____
____
____
____

Notes

Daily Tracking

DATE:

S M T W T F S

Fluid Tracker: 8 oz | 8 oz | 8 oz | 8 oz | 8 oz | 8 oz | 8 oz | 8 oz

Meal Tracking

Time	Meal	Pain Scale 0-5 0= No pain 5= Severe
BREAKFAST		
LUNCH		
DINNER		
SNACKS		

Bowel Activity

Normal	Very Hard	Abnormalities
		☐ Blood ☐ Mucus ☐ Other ______
		☐ Blood ☐ Mucus ☐ Other ______
		☐ Blood ☐ Mucus ☐ Other ______
		☐ Blood ☐ Mucus ☐ Other ______
	More?	

Other Symptoms

☐ Bloating ☐ Fatigue
☐ Nausea ☐ Flatulence
☐ Vomiting
☐ Other ______________________

Stress Level

Sleep

Energy Level

Activity Level

Pain Location (If Applicable)

☐ Abdomen ☐ Joints
☐ Stomach ☐ Rectum
☐ Other ______________________

Medications

____
____
____
____
____

Notes

Daily Tracking

DATE:

S M T W T F S

Fluid Tracker: 8 oz | 8 oz | 8 oz | 8 oz | 8 oz | 8 oz | 8 oz | 8 oz

Meal Tracking

Time	Meal	Pain Scale 0-5 0= No pain 5= Severe
BREAKFAST		
LUNCH		
DINNER		
SNACKS		

Bowel Activity

Normal	Very Hard	Abnormalities
		☐ Blood ☐ Mucus ☐ Other ______
		☐ Blood ☐ Mucus ☐ Other ______
		☐ Blood ☐ Mucus ☐ Other ______
		☐ Blood ☐ Mucus ☐ Other ______
	More?	

Other Symptoms

☐ Bloating ☐ Fatigue
☐ Nausea ☐ Flatulence
☐ Vomiting
☐ Other ______

Stress Level

Sleep

Energy Level

Activity Level

Pain Location (If Applicable)

☐ Abdomen ☐ Joints
☐ Stomach ☐ Rectum
☐ Other ______

Medications

______
______
______
______
______

Notes

Daily Tracking

DATE:

S M T W T F S

Fluid Tracker: 8 oz | 8 oz | 8 oz | 8 oz | 8 oz | 8 oz | 8 oz | 8 oz

Meal Tracking

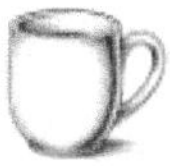

Time	Meal	Pain Scale 0-5 0= No pain 5= Severe
BREAKFAST		
LUNCH		
DINNER		
SNACKS		

Bowel Activity

Normal	Very Hard	Abnormalities
		☐ Blood ☐ Mucus ☐ Other ______
		☐ Blood ☐ Mucus ☐ Other ______
		☐ Blood ☐ Mucus ☐ Other ______
		☐ Blood ☐ Mucus ☐ Other ______
	More?	

Other Symptoms

- ☐ Bloating
- ☐ Fatigue
- ☐ Nausea
- ☐ Flatulence
- ☐ Vomiting
- ☐ Other ______________________

Stress Level

Sleep

Energy Level

Activity Level

Pain Location (If Applicable)

- ☐ Abdomen
- ☐ Joints
- ☐ Stomach
- ☐ Rectum
- ☐ Other ______________________

Medications

____

____

____

____

____

Notes

Weekly Reflections

What was the best thing that happened this week?

What was the hardest thing that happened this week?

What helped you the most this week?

What gave you hope this week?

What's one small win you can celebrate?

Was there something that eased your stress?

Overall, this week I felt

☐ A little better ☐ A lot better ☐ A little worse ☐ A lot worse

☐ About the same

Next week I want to:

____

____

____

____

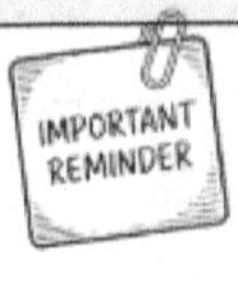

Sometimes the bravest act is simply showing up. You've done that today.

Daily Tracking

DATE:

S M T W T F S

Fluid Tracker 8 oz 8 oz 8 oz 8 oz 8 oz 8 oz 8 oz 8 oz

Meal Tracking

Time	Meal	Pain Scale 0-5 0= No pain 5= Severe
BREAKFAST		
LUNCH		
DINNER		
SNACKS		

Bowel Activity

Normal	Very Hard	Abnormalities
		☐ Blood ☐ Mucus ☐ Other ____
		☐ Blood ☐ Mucus ☐ Other ____
		☐ Blood ☐ Mucus ☐ Other ____
		☐ Blood ☐ Mucus ☐ Other ____
	More?	

Other Symptoms

☐ Bloating ☐ Fatigue
☐ Nausea ☐ Flatulence
☐ Vomiting
☐ Other ____________________

Stress Level

Sleep

Energy Level

Activity Level

Pain Location (If Applicable)

☐ Abdomen ☐ Joints
☐ Stomach ☐ Rectum
☐ Other ____________________

Medications

____
____
____
____
____

Notes

Daily Tracking

DATE:

S M T W T F S

Fluid Tracker 8 oz 8 oz 8 oz 8 oz 8 oz 8 oz 8 oz 8 oz

Meal Tracking

Time	Meal	Pain Scale 0-5 0= No pain 5= Severe
BREAKFAST		
LUNCH		
DINNER		
SNACKS		

Bowel Activity

Normal	Very Hard	Abnormalities
		☐ Blood ☐ Mucus ☐ Other ________
		☐ Blood ☐ Mucus ☐ Other ________
		☐ Blood ☐ Mucus ☐ Other ________
		☐ Blood ☐ Mucus ☐ Other ________
	More?	

Other Symptoms

- ☐ Bloating
- ☐ Fatigue
- ☐ Nausea
- ☐ Flatulence
- ☐ Vomiting
- ☐ Other ______________________

Stress Level

Sleep

Energy Level

Activity Level

Pain Location (If Applicable)

- ☐ Abdomen
- ☐ Joints
- ☐ Stomach
- ☐ Rectum
- ☐ Other ______________________

Notes

Medications

____

____

____

____

____

Daily Tracking

DATE:

S M T W T F S

Meal Tracking

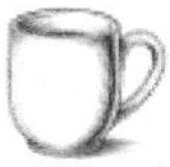

Fluid Tracker: 8 oz | 8 oz | 8 oz | 8 oz | 8 oz | 8 oz | 8 oz | 8 oz

Time	Meal	Pain Scale 0-5 0= No pain 5= Severe
BREAKFAST		
LUNCH		
DINNER		
SNACKS		

Bowel Activity

Normal	Very Hard	Abnormalities
		☐ Blood ☐ Mucus ☐ Other ____
		☐ Blood ☐ Mucus ☐ Other ____
		☐ Blood ☐ Mucus ☐ Other ____
		☐ Blood ☐ Mucus ☐ Other ____
	More?	

Other Symptoms

☐ Bloating ☐ Fatigue
☐ Nausea ☐ Flatulence
☐ Vomiting
☐ Other ____________________

Stress Level

Sleep

Energy Level

Activity Level

Pain Location (If Applicable)

☐ Abdomen ☐ Joints
☐ Stomach ☐ Rectum
☐ Other ____________________

Medications

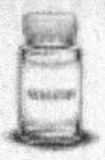

____
____
____
____
____

Notes

Daily Tracking

DATE:

S M T W T F S

Meal Tracking

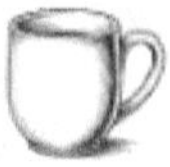

Fluid Tracker 8 oz 8 oz 8 oz 8 oz 8 oz 8 oz 8 oz 8 oz

Time	Meal	Pain Scale 0-5 0= No pain 5= Severe
BREAKFAST		
LUNCH		
DINNER		
SNACKS		

Bowel Activity

Normal	Very Hard	Abnormalities
		☐ Blood ☐ Mucus ☐ Other ______
		☐ Blood ☐ Mucus ☐ Other ______
		☐ Blood ☐ Mucus ☐ Other ______
		☐ Blood ☐ Mucus ☐ Other ______
	More?	

Other Symptoms

☐ Bloating ☐ Fatigue
☐ Nausea ☐ Flatulence
☐ Vomiting
☐ Other ______________________

Stress Level

Sleep

Energy Level

Activity Level

Pain Location (If Applicable)

☐ Abdomen ☐ Joints
☐ Stomach ☐ Rectum
☐ Other ______________________

Medications

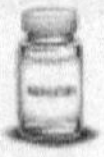

____
____
____
____
____

Notes

Daily Tracking

DATE:

S M T W T F S

Fluid Tracker: 8 oz | 8 oz | 8 oz | 8 oz | 8 oz | 8 oz | 8 oz | 8 oz

Meal Tracking

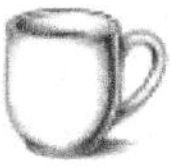

Time	Meal	Pain Scale 0-5 0= No pain 5= Severe
BREAKFAST		
LUNCH		
DINNER		
SNACKS		

Bowel Activity

Normal	Very Hard	Abnormalities
		☐ Blood ☐ Mucus ☐ Other ______
		☐ Blood ☐ Mucus ☐ Other ______
		☐ Blood ☐ Mucus ☐ Other ______
		☐ Blood ☐ Mucus ☐ Other ______
	More?	

Other Symptoms

- ☐ Bloating
- ☐ Fatigue
- ☐ Nausea
- ☐ Flatulence
- ☐ Vomiting
- ☐ Other ______________________

Stress Level

Sleep

Energy Level

Activity Level

Pain Location (If Applicable)

- ☐ Abdomen
- ☐ Joints
- ☐ Stomach
- ☐ Rectum
- ☐ Other ______________________

Notes

Medications

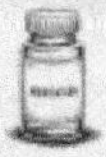

____

____

____

____

____

Daily Tracking

DATE:

S M T W T F S

Fluid Tracker: 8 oz | 8 oz | 8 oz | 8 oz | 8 oz | 8 oz | 8 oz | 8 oz

Meal Tracking

Time	Meal	Pain Scale 0-5 0= No pain 5= Severe
BREAKFAST		
LUNCH		
DINNER		
SNACKS		

Bowel Activity

Normal	Very Hard	Abnormalities
		☐ Blood ☐ Mucus ☐ Other ______
		☐ Blood ☐ Mucus ☐ Other ______
		☐ Blood ☐ Mucus ☐ Other ______
		☐ Blood ☐ Mucus ☐ Other ______
	More?	

Other Symptoms

☐ Bloating ☐ Fatigue
☐ Nausea ☐ Flatulence
☐ Vomiting
☐ Other ______________________

Stress Level

Sleep

Energy Level

Activity Level

Pain Location (If Applicable)

☐ Abdomen ☐ Joints
☐ Stomach ☐ Rectum
☐ Other ______________________

Medications

____
____
____
____
____

Notes

Daily Tracking

DATE:

S M T W T F S

Fluid Tracker: 8 oz | 8 oz | 8 oz | 8 oz | 8 oz | 8 oz | 8 oz | 8 oz

Meal Tracking

Time	Meal	Pain Scale 0-5 0= No pain 5= Severe
BREAKFAST		
LUNCH		
DINNER		
SNACKS		

Bowel Activity

Normal	Very Hard	Abnormalities
		☐ Blood ☐ Mucus ☐ Other ______
		☐ Blood ☐ Mucus ☐ Other ______
		☐ Blood ☐ Mucus ☐ Other ______
		☐ Blood ☐ Mucus ☐ Other ______
	More?	

Other Symptoms

☐ Bloating ☐ Fatigue
☐ Nausea ☐ Flatulence
☐ Vomiting
☐ Other ______________________

Stress Level

Sleep

Energy Level

Activity Level

Pain Location (If Applicable)

☐ Abdomen ☐ Joints
☐ Stomach ☐ Rectum
☐ Other ______________________

Medications

____
____
____
____
____

Notes

Weekly Reflections

What was the best thing that happened this week?

What was the hardest thing that happened this week?

What helped you the most this week?

What gave you hope this week?

What's one small win you can celebrate?

Was there something that eased your stress?

Overall, this week I felt

☐ A little better ☐ A lot better ☐ A little worse ☐ A lot worse

☐ About the same

Next week I want to:

____

____

____

____

Gratitude can be quiet. Notice one small thing that made this week lighter.

Daily Tracking

DATE:	S M T W T F S

Fluid Tracker 8 oz 8 oz 8 oz 8 oz 8 oz 8 oz 8 oz 8 oz

Meal Tracking

Time	Meal	Pain Scale 0-5 0= No pain 5= Severe
BREAKFAST		
LUNCH		
DINNER		
SNACKS		

Bowel Activity

Normal	Very Hard	Abnormalities
		☐ Blood ☐ Mucus ☐ Other ______
		☐ Blood ☐ Mucus ☐ Other ______
		☐ Blood ☐ Mucus ☐ Other ______
		☐ Blood ☐ Mucus ☐ Other ______
	More?	

Other Symptoms

- ☐ Bloating
- ☐ Fatigue
- ☐ Nausea
- ☐ Flatulence
- ☐ Vomiting
- ☐ Other ______________________

Stress Level

Sleep

Energy Level

Activity Level

Pain Location (If Applicable)

- ☐ Abdomen
- ☐ Joints
- ☐ Stomach
- ☐ Rectum
- ☐ Other ______________________

Notes

Medications

____

____

____

____

____

Daily Tracking

DATE:

S M T W T F S

Meal Tracking

Fluid Tracker 8 oz 8 oz 8 oz 8 oz 8 oz 8 oz 8 oz 8 oz

Time	Meal	Pain Scale 0-5 0= No pain 5= Severe
BREAKFAST		
LUNCH		
DINNER		
SNACKS		

Bowel Activity

Normal	Very Hard	Abnormalities
		☐ Blood ☐ Mucus ☐ Other ______
		☐ Blood ☐ Mucus ☐ Other ______
		☐ Blood ☐ Mucus ☐ Other ______
		☐ Blood ☐ Mucus ☐ Other ______
	More?	

Other Symptoms

☐ Bloating ☐ Fatigue
☐ Nausea ☐ Flatulence
☐ Vomiting
☐ Other ______________________

Stress Level

Sleep

Energy Level

Activity Level

Pain Location (If Applicable)

☐ Abdomen ☐ Joints
☐ Stomach ☐ Rectum
☐ Other ______________________

Medications

____
____
____
____
____

Notes

Daily Tracking

DATE:

S M T W T F S

Fluid Tracker 8 oz 8 oz 8 oz 8 oz 8 oz 8 oz 8 oz 8 oz

leal Tracking

Time	Meal	Pain Scale 0-5 0= No pain 5= Severe
3REAKFAST		
.UNCH		
)INNER		
5NACKS		

3owel Activity

Normal	Very Hard	Abnormalities
		☐ Blood ☐ Mucus ☐ Other ______
		☐ Blood ☐ Mucus ☐ Other ______
		☐ Blood ☐ Mucus ☐ Other ______
		☐ Blood ☐ Mucus ☐ Other ______
	More?	

Other Symptoms

☐ Bloating ☐ Fatigue
☐ Nausea ☐ Flatulence
☐ Vomiting
☐ Other ______________________

Stress Level

Sleep

Energy Level

Activity Level

Pain Location (If Applicable)

☐ Abdomen ☐ Joints
☐ Stomach ☐ Rectum
☐ Other ______________________

Medications

____
____
____
____
____

Iotes

Daily Tracking

DATE:

S M T W T F S

Fluid Tracker 8 oz 8 oz 8 oz 8 oz 8 oz 8 oz 8 oz 8 oz

Meal Tracking

Time	Meal	Pain Scale 0-5 0= No pain 5= Severe
BREAKFAST		
LUNCH		
DINNER		
SNACKS		

Bowel Activity

Normal	Very Hard	Abnormalities
		☐ Blood ☐ Mucus ☐ Other ______
		☐ Blood ☐ Mucus ☐ Other ______
		☐ Blood ☐ Mucus ☐ Other ______
		☐ Blood ☐ Mucus ☐ Other ______
	More?	

Other Symptoms

☐ Bloating ☐ Fatigue
☐ Nausea ☐ Flatulence
☐ Vomiting
☐ Other ______________________

Stress Level

Sleep

Energy Level

Activity Level

Pain Location (If Applicable)

☐ Abdomen ☐ Joints
☐ Stomach ☐ Rectum
☐ Other ______________________

Medications

____
____
____
____
____

Notes

Daily Tracking

DATE:

S M T W T F S

Fluid Tracker: 8 oz | 8 oz | 8 oz | 8 oz | 8 oz | 8 oz | 8 oz | 8 oz

Meal Tracking

Time	Meal	Pain Scale 0-5 0= No pain 5= Severe
BREAKFAST		
LUNCH		
DINNER		
SNACKS		

Bowel Activity

Normal	Very Hard	Abnormalities
		☐ Blood ☐ Mucus ☐ Other ____
		☐ Blood ☐ Mucus ☐ Other ____
		☐ Blood ☐ Mucus ☐ Other ____
		☐ Blood ☐ Mucus ☐ Other ____
	More?	

Other Symptoms

☐ Bloating ☐ Fatigue
☐ Nausea ☐ Flatulence
☐ Vomiting
☐ Other ____________________

Stress Level

Sleep

Energy Level

Activity Level

Pain Location (If Applicable)

☐ Abdomen ☐ Joints
☐ Stomach ☐ Rectum
☐ Other ____________________

Medications

____
____
____
____
____

Notes

Daily Tracking

DATE:

S M T W T F S

Meal Tracking

Fluid Tracker: 8 oz | 8 oz | 8 oz | 8 oz | 8 oz | 8 oz | 8 oz | 8 oz

Time	Meal	Pain Scale 0-5 0= No pain 5= Severe
BREAKFAST		
LUNCH		
DINNER		
SNACKS		

Bowel Activity

Normal	Very Hard	Abnormalities
		☐ Blood ☐ Mucus ☐ Other ______
		☐ Blood ☐ Mucus ☐ Other ______
		☐ Blood ☐ Mucus ☐ Other ______
		☐ Blood ☐ Mucus ☐ Other ______
	More?	

Other Symptoms

☐ Bloating ☐ Fatigue
☐ Nausea ☐ Flatulence
☐ Vomiting
☐ Other ______________________

Stress Level

Sleep

Energy Level

Activity Level

Pain Location (If Applicable)

☐ Abdomen ☐ Joints
☐ Stomach ☐ Rectum
☐ Other ______________________

Medications

____
____
____
____
____

Notes

Daily Tracking

DATE:

S M T W T F S

Fluid Tracker: 8 oz | 8 oz | 8 oz | 8 oz | 8 oz | 8 oz | 8 oz | 8 oz

Meal Tracking

Time	Meal	Pain Scale 0-5 0= No pain 5= Severe
BREAKFAST		
LUNCH		
DINNER		
SNACKS		

Bowel Activity

Normal	Very Hard	Abnormalities
		☐ Blood ☐ Mucus ☐ Other ______
		☐ Blood ☐ Mucus ☐ Other ______
		☐ Blood ☐ Mucus ☐ Other ______
		☐ Blood ☐ Mucus ☐ Other ______
	More?	

Other Symptoms

☐ Bloating ☐ Fatigue
☐ Nausea ☐ Flatulence
☐ Vomiting
☐ Other ______________________

Stress Level

Sleep

Energy Level

Activity Level

Pain Location (If Applicable)

☐ Abdomen ☐ Joints
☐ Stomach ☐ Rectum
☐ Other ______________________

Medications

____
____
____
____
____

Notes

Weekly Reflections

What was the best thing that happened this week?

What was the hardest thing that happened this week?

What helped you the most this week?

What gave you hope this week?

What's one small win you can celebrate?

Was there something that eased your stress?

Overall, this week I felt

☐ A little better ☐ A lot better ☐ A little worse ☐ A lot worse

☐ About the same

Next week I want to:

____

____

____

____

You are not alone on this journey. Countless others walk alongside you in spirit.

Monthly Thoughts

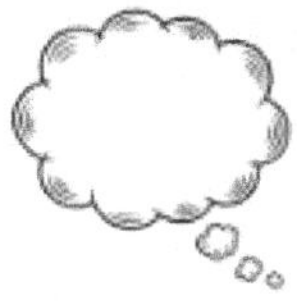

This page is your space to step back and see the bigger picture. Each month brings its own challenges and small victories—use this space to notice patterns, celebrate progress, and reflect on what your body and mind are teaching you. These notes can guide you forward with greater clarity and self-compassion.

This Month I Noticed...

(Write down patterns in your symptoms, energy, or mood.)

Biggest Challenge: ______________________________

____

Brightest Moment: ______________________________

____

Triggers I Noticed: ______________________________

____

Things That Helped: ______________________________

____

Medication / Treatment Notes: (Any changes, side effects, or adjustments.) ______________________________

____

____

Self-Care Check-In

How well I cared for myself this month: ______________________________

____

Looking Forward

Next month I want to focus on: ______________________________

____

____

Symptom Overview

Good Days: ________ Mild Days: ________ Flare Days: ________

Be proud of the care you've given yourself this far.

Daily Tracking

DATE:

S M T W T F S

Fluid Tracker: 8 oz | 8 oz | 8 oz | 8 oz | 8 oz | 8 oz | 8 oz | 8 oz

Meal Tracking

Time	Meal	Pain Scale 0-5 0= No pain 5= Severe
BREAKFAST		
LUNCH		
DINNER		
SNACKS		

Bowel Activity

Normal	Very Hard	Abnormalities
		☐ Blood ☐ Mucus ☐ Other ____
		☐ Blood ☐ Mucus ☐ Other ____
		☐ Blood ☐ Mucus ☐ Other ____
		☐ Blood ☐ Mucus ☐ Other ____
	More?	

Other Symptoms

- ☐ Bloating
- ☐ Nausea
- ☐ Vomiting
- ☐ Fatigue
- ☐ Flatulence
- ☐ Other ____________________

Stress Level

Sleep

Energy Level

Activity Level

Pain Location (If Applicable)

- ☐ Abdomen
- ☐ Stomach
- ☐ Joints
- ☐ Rectum
- ☐ Other ____________________

Medications

____

____

____

____

____

Notes

Daily Tracking

DATE:

S M T W T F S

Fluid Tracker: 8 oz | 8 oz | 8 oz | 8 oz | 8 oz | 8 oz | 8 oz | 8 oz

Meal Tracking

Time	Meal	Pain Scale 0-5 0= No pain 5= Severe
BREAKFAST		
LUNCH		
DINNER		
SNACKS		

Bowel Activity

Normal	Very Hard	Abnormalities
		☐ Blood ☐ Mucus ☐ Other ______
		☐ Blood ☐ Mucus ☐ Other ______
		☐ Blood ☐ Mucus ☐ Other ______
		☐ Blood ☐ Mucus ☐ Other ______
	More?	

Other Symptoms

☐ Bloating ☐ Fatigue
☐ Nausea ☐ Flatulence
☐ Vomiting
☐ Other ______________________

Stress Level

Sleep

Energy Level

Activity Level

Pain Location (If Applicable)

☐ Abdomen ☐ Joints
☐ Stomach ☐ Rectum
☐ Other ______________________

Medications

____
____
____
____
____

Notes

Daily Tracking

DATE: ____________________

S M T W T F S

Fluid Tracker: 8 oz | 8 oz | 8 oz | 8 oz | 8 oz | 8 oz | 8 oz | 8 oz

Meal Tracking

Time	Meal	Pain Scale 0-5 0= No pain 5= Severe
BREAKFAST		
LUNCH		
DINNER		
SNACKS		

Bowel Activity

Normal	Very Hard	Abnormalities
		☐ Blood ☐ Mucus ☐ Other ______
		☐ Blood ☐ Mucus ☐ Other ______
		☐ Blood ☐ Mucus ☐ Other ______
		☐ Blood ☐ Mucus ☐ Other ______
	More?	

Other Symptoms

☐ Bloating ☐ Fatigue
☐ Nausea ☐ Flatulence
☐ Vomiting
☐ Other ____________________

Stress Level

Sleep

Energy Level

Activity Level

Pain Location (If Applicable)

☐ Abdomen ☐ Joints
☐ Stomach ☐ Rectum
☐ Other ____________________

Medications

____
____
____
____
____

Notes

Daily Tracking

DATE:

S M T W T F S

Fluid Tracker 8 oz 8 oz 8 oz 8 oz 8 oz 8 oz 8 oz 8 oz

Meal Tracking

Time	Meal	Pain Scale 0-5 0= No pain 5= Severe
BREAKFAST		
LUNCH		
DINNER		
SNACKS		

Bowel Activity

Normal	Very Hard	Abnormalities
		☐ Blood ☐ Mucus ☐ Other ______
		☐ Blood ☐ Mucus ☐ Other ______
		☐ Blood ☐ Mucus ☐ Other ______
		☐ Blood ☐ Mucus ☐ Other ______
	More?	

Other Symptoms

☐ Bloating ☐ Fatigue
☐ Nausea ☐ Flatulence
☐ Vomiting
☐ Other ____________________

Stress Level

Sleep

Energy Level

Activity Level

Pain Location (If Applicable)

☐ Abdomen ☐ Joints
☐ Stomach ☐ Rectum
☐ Other ____________________

Notes

Medications

____
____
____
____
____

Daily Tracking

DATE:

S M T W T F S

Fluid Tracker: 8 oz | 8 oz | 8 oz | 8 oz | 8 oz | 8 oz | 8 oz | 8 oz

Meal Tracking

Time	Meal	Pain Scale 0-5 0= No pain 5= Severe
BREAKFAST		
LUNCH		
DINNER		
SNACKS		

Bowel Activity

Normal	Very Hard	Abnormalities
		☐ Blood ☐ Mucus ☐ Other ________
		☐ Blood ☐ Mucus ☐ Other ________
		☐ Blood ☐ Mucus ☐ Other ________
		☐ Blood ☐ Mucus ☐ Other ________
	More?	

Pain Location (If Applicable)

☐ Abdomen ☐ Joints
☐ Stomach ☐ Rectum
☐ Other ____________________

Notes

Other Symptoms

☐ Bloating ☐ Fatigue
☐ Nausea ☐ Flatulence
☐ Vomiting
☐ Other ____________________

Stress Level

Sleep

Energy Level

Activity Level

Medications

____
____
____
____
____

Daily Tracking

DATE:

S M T W T F S

Fluid Tracker: 8 oz | 8 oz | 8 oz | 8 oz | 8 oz | 8 oz | 8 oz | 8 oz

Meal Tracking

Time	Meal	Pain Scale 0-5 0= No pain 5= Severe
BREAKFAST		
LUNCH		
DINNER		
SNACKS		

Bowel Activity

Normal	Very Hard	Abnormalities
		☐ Blood ☐ Mucus ☐ Other ______
		☐ Blood ☐ Mucus ☐ Other ______
		☐ Blood ☐ Mucus ☐ Other ______
		☐ Blood ☐ Mucus ☐ Other ______
	More?	

Other Symptoms

☐ Bloating ☐ Fatigue
☐ Nausea ☐ Flatulence
☐ Vomiting
☐ Other ____________________

Stress Level

Sleep

Energy Level

Activity Level

Pain Location (If Applicable)

☐ Abdomen ☐ Joints
☐ Stomach ☐ Rectum
☐ Other ____________________

Medications

____
____
____
____
____

Notes

Daily Tracking

DATE:

S M T W T F S

Fluid Tracker 8 oz 8 oz 8 oz 8 oz 8 oz 8 oz 8 oz 8 oz

Meal Tracking

Time	Meal	Pain Scale 0-5 0= No pain 5= Severe
BREAKFAST		
LUNCH		
DINNER		
SNACKS		

Bowel Activity

Normal	Very Hard	Abnormalities
		☐ Blood ☐ Mucus ☐ Other ______
		☐ Blood ☐ Mucus ☐ Other ______
		☐ Blood ☐ Mucus ☐ Other ______
		☐ Blood ☐ Mucus ☐ Other ______
	More?	

Other Symptoms

☐ Bloating ☐ Fatigue
☐ Nausea ☐ Flatulence
☐ Vomiting
☐ Other ______

Stress Level

Sleep

Energy Level

Activity Leve

Pain Location (If Applicable)

☐ Abdomen ☐ Joints
☐ Stomach ☐ Rectum
☐ Other ______

Medications

______
______
______
______
______

Notes

Weekly Reflections

What was the best thing that happened this week?

What was the hardest thing that happened this week?

What helped you the most this week?

What gave you hope this week?

What's one small win you can celebrate?

Was there something that eased your stress?

Overall, this week I felt

☐ A little better ☐ A lot better ☐ A little worse ☐ A lot worse
☐ About the same

Next week I want to:

____

____

____

____

Even when the path is hard, your resilience shines. Keep going, gently.

Daily Tracking

DATE:

S M T W T F S

Fluid Tracker: 8 oz | 8 oz | 8 oz | 8 oz | 8 oz | 8 oz | 8 oz | 8 oz

Meal Tracking

Time	Meal	Pain Scale 0-5 0= No pain 5= Severe
BREAKFAST		
LUNCH		
DINNER		
SNACKS		

Bowel Activity

Normal	Very Hard	Abnormalities
		☐ Blood ☐ Mucus ☐ Other ____
		☐ Blood ☐ Mucus ☐ Other ____
		☐ Blood ☐ Mucus ☐ Other ____
		☐ Blood ☐ Mucus ☐ Other ____
	More?	

Other Symptoms

- ☐ Bloating
- ☐ Fatigue
- ☐ Nausea
- ☐ Flatulence
- ☐ Vomiting
- ☐ Other ____________________

Stress Level

Sleep

Energy Level

Activity Level

Pain Location (If Applicable)

- ☐ Abdomen
- ☐ Joints
- ☐ Stomach
- ☐ Rectum
- ☐ Other ____________________

Medications

____

____

____

____

____

Notes

Daily Tracking

DATE: ____________________

S M T W T F S

Fluid Tracker: 8 oz | 8 oz | 8 oz | 8 oz | 8 oz | 8 oz | 8 oz | 8 oz

Meal Tracking

Time	Meal	Pain Scale 0-5 0= No pain 5= Severe
BREAKFAST		
LUNCH		
DINNER		
SNACKS		

Bowel Activity

Normal	Very Hard	Abnormalities
		☐ Blood ☐ Mucus ☐ Other ______
		☐ Blood ☐ Mucus ☐ Other ______
		☐ Blood ☐ Mucus ☐ Other ______
		☐ Blood ☐ Mucus ☐ Other ______
	More?	

Other Symptoms

- ☐ Bloating
- ☐ Fatigue
- ☐ Nausea
- ☐ Flatulence
- ☐ Vomiting
- ☐ Other ____________________

Stress Level

Sleep

Energy Level

Activity Level

Pain Location (If Applicable)

- ☐ Abdomen
- ☐ Joints
- ☐ Stomach
- ☐ Rectum
- ☐ Other ____________________

Medications

____

____

____

____

____

Notes

Daily Tracking

DATE:

S M T W T F S

Fluid Tracker 8 oz 8 oz 8 oz 8 oz 8 oz 8 oz 8 oz 8 oz

Meal Tracking

Time	Meal	Pain Scale 0-5 0= No pain 5= Severe
BREAKFAST		
LUNCH		
DINNER		
SNACKS		

Bowel Activity

Normal	Very Hard	Abnormalities
		☐ Blood ☐ Mucus ☐ Other
		☐ Blood ☐ Mucus ☐ Other
		☐ Blood ☐ Mucus ☐ Other
		☐ Blood ☐ Mucus ☐ Other
	More?	

Other Symptoms

☐ Bloating ☐ Fatigue
☐ Nausea ☐ Flatulence
☐ Vomiting
☐ Other ______________________

Stress Level

Sleep

Energy Level

Activity Level

Pain Location (If Applicable)

☐ Abdomen ☐ Joints
☐ Stomach ☐ Rectum
☐ Other ______________________

Medications

Notes

Daily Tracking

DATE:

S M T W T F S

Fluid Tracker 8 oz 8 oz 8 oz 8 oz 8 oz 8 oz 8 oz 8 oz

Meal Tracking

Time	Meal	Pain Scale 0-5 0= No pain 5= Severe
BREAKFAST		
LUNCH		
DINNER		
SNACKS		

Bowel Activity

Normal	Very Hard	Abnormalities
		☐ Blood ☐ Mucus ☐ Other ____
		☐ Blood ☐ Mucus ☐ Other ____
		☐ Blood ☐ Mucus ☐ Other ____
		☐ Blood ☐ Mucus ☐ Other ____
	More?	

Other Symptoms

☐ Bloating ☐ Fatigue
☐ Nausea ☐ Flatulence
☐ Vomiting
☐ Other ______________________

Stress Level

Sleep

Energy Level

Activity Level

Pain Location (If Applicable)

☐ Abdomen ☐ Joints
☐ Stomach ☐ Rectum
☐ Other ______________________

Notes

Medications

____

____

____

____

____

Daily Tracking

DATE:

S M T W T F S

Fluid Tracker: 8 oz | 8 oz | 8 oz | 8 oz | 8 oz | 8 oz | 8 oz | 8 oz

Meal Tracking

Time	Meal	Pain Scale 0-5 0= No pain 5= Severe
BREAKFAST		
LUNCH		
DINNER		
SNACKS		

Bowel Activity

Normal	Very Hard	Abnormalities
		☐ Blood ☐ Mucus ☐ Other ______
		☐ Blood ☐ Mucus ☐ Other ______
		☐ Blood ☐ Mucus ☐ Other ______
		☐ Blood ☐ Mucus ☐ Other ______
	More?	

Other Symptoms

☐ Bloating ☐ Fatigue
☐ Nausea ☐ Flatulence
☐ Vomiting
☐ Other ______________________

Stress Level

Sleep

Energy Level

Activity Level

Pain Location (If Applicable)

☐ Abdomen ☐ Joints
☐ Stomach ☐ Rectum
☐ Other ______________________

Medications

____
____
____
____
____

Notes

Daily Tracking

DATE:

S M T W T F S

Fluid Tracker: 8 oz | 8 oz | 8 oz | 8 oz | 8 oz | 8 oz | 8 oz | 8 oz

Meal Tracking

Time	Meal	Pain Scale 0-5 0= No pain 5= Severe
BREAKFAST		
LUNCH		
DINNER		
SNACKS		

Bowel Activity

Normal	Very Hard	Abnormalities
		☐ Blood ☐ Mucus ☐ Other ____
		☐ Blood ☐ Mucus ☐ Other ____
		☐ Blood ☐ Mucus ☐ Other ____
		☐ Blood ☐ Mucus ☐ Other ____
	More?	

Other Symptoms

☐ Bloating ☐ Fatigue
☐ Nausea ☐ Flatulence
☐ Vomiting
☐ Other ____________________

Stress Level

Sleep

Energy Level

Activity Level

Pain Location (If Applicable)

☐ Abdomen ☐ Joints
☐ Stomach ☐ Rectum
☐ Other ____________________

Medications

____
____
____
____
____

Notes

Daily Tracking

DATE:

S M T W T F S

Fluid Tracker: 8 oz | 8 oz | 8 oz | 8 oz | 8 oz | 8 oz | 8 oz | 8 oz

Meal Tracking

Time	Meal	Pain Scale 0-5 0= No pain 5= Severe
BREAKFAST		
LUNCH		
DINNER		
SNACKS		

Bowel Activity

Normal	Very Hard	Abnormalities
		☐ Blood ☐ Mucus ☐ Other ______
		☐ Blood ☐ Mucus ☐ Other ______
		☐ Blood ☐ Mucus ☐ Other ______
		☐ Blood ☐ Mucus ☐ Other ______
	More?	

Other Symptoms

☐ Bloating ☐ Fatigue
☐ Nausea ☐ Flatulence
☐ Vomiting
☐ Other ______________________

Stress Level

Sleep

Energy Level

Activity Level

Pain Location (If Applicable)

☐ Abdomen ☐ Joints
☐ Stomach ☐ Rectum
☐ Other ______________________

Medications

____
____
____
____
____

Notes

Weekly Reflections

What was the best thing that happened this week?

What was the hardest thing that happened this week?

What helped you the most this week?

What gave you hope this week?

What's one small win you can celebrate?

Was there something that eased your stress?

Overall, this week I felt

☐ A little better ☐ A lot better ☐ A little worse ☐ A lot worse

☐ About the same

Next week I want to:

____

____

____

____

IMPORTANT REMINDER

Look back at how far you've come. Each page shows your persistence and care.

Daily Tracking

DATE:

S M T W T F S

Fluid Tracker 8 oz 8 oz 8 oz 8 oz 8 oz 8 oz 8 oz 8 oz

Meal Tracking

Time	Meal	Pain Scale 0-5 0= No pain 5= Severe
BREAKFAST		
LUNCH		
DINNER		
SNACKS		

Bowel Activity

Normal	Very Hard	Abnormalities
		☐ Blood ☐ Mucus ☐ Other ____
		☐ Blood ☐ Mucus ☐ Other ____
		☐ Blood ☐ Mucus ☐ Other ____
		☐ Blood ☐ Mucus ☐ Other ____
	More?	

Other Symptoms

- ☐ Bloating
- ☐ Fatigue
- ☐ Nausea
- ☐ Flatulence
- ☐ Vomiting
- ☐ Other ____________________

Stress Level

Sleep

Energy Level

Activity Level

Pain Location (If Applicable)

- ☐ Abdomen
- ☐ Joints
- ☐ Stomach
- ☐ Rectum
- ☐ Other ____________________

Medications

____

____

____

____

____

Notes

Daily Tracking

DATE:

S M T W T F S

Fluid Tracker: 8 oz | 8 oz | 8 oz | 8 oz | 8 oz | 8 oz | 8 oz | 8 oz

Meal Tracking

Time	Meal	Pain Scale 0-5 0= No pain 5= Severe
BREAKFAST		
LUNCH		
DINNER		
SNACKS		

Bowel Activity

Normal	Very Hard	Abnormalities
		☐ Blood ☐ Mucus ☐ Other ________
		☐ Blood ☐ Mucus ☐ Other ________
		☐ Blood ☐ Mucus ☐ Other ________
		☐ Blood ☐ Mucus ☐ Other ________
	More?	

Other Symptoms

☐ Bloating ☐ Fatigue
☐ Nausea ☐ Flatulence
☐ Vomiting
☐ Other ____________________

Stress Level

Sleep

Energy Level

Activity Level

Pain Location (If Applicable)

☐ Abdomen ☐ Joints
☐ Stomach ☐ Rectum
☐ Other ____________________

Medications

____
____
____
____
____

Notes

Daily Tracking

DATE:

S M T W T F S

Fluid Tracker 8 oz 8 oz 8 oz 8 oz 8 oz 8 oz 8 oz 8 oz

Meal Tracking

Time	Meal	Pain Scale 0-5 0= No pain 5= Severe
BREAKFAST		
LUNCH		
DINNER		
SNACKS		

Bowel Activity

Normal	Very Hard	Abnormalities
		☐ Blood ☐ Mucus ☐ Other ______
		☐ Blood ☐ Mucus ☐ Other ______
		☐ Blood ☐ Mucus ☐ Other ______
		☐ Blood ☐ Mucus ☐ Other ______
	More?	

Other Symptoms

☐ Bloating ☐ Fatigue
☐ Nausea ☐ Flatulence
☐ Vomiting
☐ Other ______________________

Stress Level

Sleep

Energy Level

Activity Level

Pain Location (If Applicable)

☐ Abdomen ☐ Joints
☐ Stomach ☐ Rectum
☐ Other ______________________

Medications

____
____
____
____
____

Notes

Daily Tracking

DATE:

S M T W T F S

Fluid Tracker: 8 oz | 8 oz | 8 oz | 8 oz | 8 oz | 8 oz | 8 oz | 8 oz

Meal Tracking

Time	Meal	Pain Scale 0-5 0= No pain 5= Severe
BREAKFAST		
LUNCH		
DINNER		
SNACKS		

Bowel Activity

Normal	Very Hard	Abnormalities
		☐ Blood ☐ Mucus ☐ Other ______
		☐ Blood ☐ Mucus ☐ Other ______
		☐ Blood ☐ Mucus ☐ Other ______
		☐ Blood ☐ Mucus ☐ Other ______
	More?	

Other Symptoms

- ☐ Bloating
- ☐ Nausea
- ☐ Vomiting
- ☐ Other ______
- ☐ Fatigue
- ☐ Flatulence

Stress Level

Sleep

Energy Level

Activity Level

Pain Location (If Applicable)

- ☐ Abdomen
- ☐ Stomach
- ☐ Other ______
- ☐ Joints
- ☐ Rectum

Notes

Medications

______
______
______
______
______

Daily Tracking

DATE:

S M T W T F S

Fluid Tracker: 8 oz | 8 oz | 8 oz | 8 oz | 8 oz | 8 oz | 8 oz | 8 oz

Meal Tracking

Time	Meal	Pain Scale 0-5 0= No pain 5= Severe
BREAKFAST		
LUNCH		
DINNER		
SNACKS		

Bowel Activity

Normal	Very Hard	Abnormalities
		☐ Blood ☐ Mucus ☐ Other ______
		☐ Blood ☐ Mucus ☐ Other ______
		☐ Blood ☐ Mucus ☐ Other ______
		☐ Blood ☐ Mucus ☐ Other ______
	More?	

Other Symptoms

- ☐ Bloating
- ☐ Fatigue
- ☐ Nausea
- ☐ Flatulence
- ☐ Vomiting
- ☐ Other ____________________

Stress Level

Sleep

Energy Level

Activity Level

Pain Location (If Applicable)

- ☐ Abdomen
- ☐ Joints
- ☐ Stomach
- ☐ Rectum
- ☐ Other ____________________

Medications

____

____

____

____

____

Notes

Daily Tracking

DATE:

S M T W T F S

Meal Tracking

Fluid Tracker: 8 oz | 8 oz | 8 oz | 8 oz | 8 oz | 8 oz | 8 oz | 8 oz

Time	Meal	Pain Scale 0-5 0= No pain 5= Severe
BREAKFAST		
LUNCH		
DINNER		
SNACKS		

Bowel Activity

Normal	Very Hard	Abnormalities
		☐ Blood ☐ Mucus ☐ Other ____
		☐ Blood ☐ Mucus ☐ Other ____
		☐ Blood ☐ Mucus ☐ Other ____
		☐ Blood ☐ Mucus ☐ Other ____
	More?	

Other Symptoms

- ☐ Bloating
- ☐ Fatigue
- ☐ Nausea
- ☐ Flatulence
- ☐ Vomiting
- ☐ Other ________________

Stress Level

Sleep

Energy Level

Activity Level

Pain Location (If Applicable)

- ☐ Abdomen
- ☐ Joints
- ☐ Stomach
- ☐ Rectum
- ☐ Other ________________

Medications

____

____

____

____

____

Notes

Daily Tracking

DATE:

S M T W T F S

Fluid Tracker 8 oz 8 oz 8 oz 8 oz 8 oz 8 oz 8 oz 8 oz

Meal Tracking

Time	Meal	Pain Scale 0-5 0= No pain 5= Severe
BREAKFAST		
LUNCH		
DINNER		
SNACKS		

Bowel Activity

Normal	Very Hard	Abnormalities
		☐ Blood ☐ Mucus ☐ Other ____
		☐ Blood ☐ Mucus ☐ Other ____
		☐ Blood ☐ Mucus ☐ Other ____
		☐ Blood ☐ Mucus ☐ Other ____
	More?	

Pain Location (If Applicable)

☐ Abdomen ☐ Joints
☐ Stomach ☐ Rectum
☐ Other ______________________

Notes

Other Symptoms

☐ Bloating ☐ Fatigue
☐ Nausea ☐ Flatulence
☐ Vomiting
☐ Other ______________________

Stress Level

Sleep

Energy Level

Activity Level

Medications

____

____

____

____

____

Weekly Reflections

What was the best thing that happened this week?

What was the hardest thing that happened this week?

What helped you the most this week?

What gave you hope this week?

What's one small win you can celebrate?

Was there something that eased your stress?

Overall, this week I felt

☐ A little better ☐ A lot better ☐ A little worse ☐ A lot worse

☐ About the same

Next week I want to:

____

____

____

____

As this chapter closes, remember: your story continues, and it's filled with hope.

Daily Tracking

DATE:

S M T W T F S

Fluid Tracker 8 oz 8 oz 8 oz 8 oz 8 oz 8 oz 8 oz 8 oz

Meal Tracking

Time	Meal	Pain Scale 0-5 0= No pain 5= Severe
BREAKFAST		
LUNCH		
DINNER		
SNACKS		

Bowel Activity

Normal	Very Hard	Abnormalities
		☐ Blood ☐ Mucus ☐ Other ______
		☐ Blood ☐ Mucus ☐ Other ______
		☐ Blood ☐ Mucus ☐ Other ______
		☐ Blood ☐ Mucus ☐ Other ______
	More?	

Other Symptoms

☐ Bloating ☐ Fatigue
☐ Nausea ☐ Flatulence
☐ Vomiting
☐ Other ______________________

Stress Level

Sleep

Energy Level

Activity Level

Pain Location (If Applicable)

☐ Abdomen ☐ Joints
☐ Stomach ☐ Rectum
☐ Other ______________________

Medications

____
____
____
____
____

Notes

Daily Tracking

DATE:

S M T W T F S

Fluid Tracker: 8 oz | 8 oz | 8 oz | 8 oz | 8 oz | 8 oz | 8 oz | 8 oz

Meal Tracking

Time	Meal	Pain Scale 0-5 0= No pain 5= Severe
BREAKFAST		
LUNCH		
DINNER		
SNACKS		

Bowel Activity

Normal	Very Hard	Abnormalities
		☐ Blood ☐ Mucus ☐ Other ______
		☐ Blood ☐ Mucus ☐ Other ______
		☐ Blood ☐ Mucus ☐ Other ______
		☐ Blood ☐ Mucus ☐ Other ______
	More?	

Other Symptoms

☐ Bloating ☐ Fatigue
☐ Nausea ☐ Flatulence
☐ Vomiting
☐ Other ______________________

Stress Level

Sleep

Energy Level

Activity Level

Pain Location (If Applicable)

☐ Abdomen ☐ Joints
☐ Stomach ☐ Rectum
☐ Other ______________________

Medications

____
____
____
____
____

Notes

Daily Tracking

DATE:

S M T W T F S

Fluid Tracker 8 oz 8 oz 8 oz 8 oz 8 oz 8 oz 8 oz 8 oz

Meal Tracking

Time	Meal	Pain Scale 0-5 0= No pain 5= Severe
BREAKFAST		
LUNCH		
DINNER		
SNACKS		

Bowel Activity

Normal	Very Hard	Abnormalities
		☐ Blood ☐ Mucus ☐ Other ______
		☐ Blood ☐ Mucus ☐ Other ______
		☐ Blood ☐ Mucus ☐ Other ______
		☐ Blood ☐ Mucus ☐ Other ______
	More?	

Pain Location (If Applicable)

- ☐ Abdomen
- ☐ Joints
- ☐ Stomach
- ☐ Rectum
- ☐ Other ______________________

Notes

Other Symptoms

- ☐ Bloating
- ☐ Fatigue
- ☐ Nausea
- ☐ Flatulence
- ☐ Vomiting
- ☐ Other ______________________

Stress Level

Sleep

Energy Level

Activity Level

Medications

____

____

____

____

____

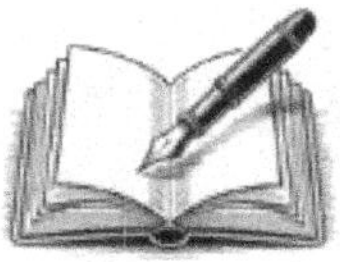

Daily Tracking

DATE: ______________________

S M T W T F S

Fluid Tracker 8 oz 8 oz 8 oz 8 oz 8 oz 8 oz 8 oz 8 oz

Meal Tracking

Time	Meal	Pain Scale 0-5 0= No pain 5= Severe
BREAKFAST		
LUNCH		
DINNER		
SNACKS		

Bowel Activity

Normal	Very Hard	Abnormalities
		☐ Blood ☐ Mucus ☐ Other ______
		☐ Blood ☐ Mucus ☐ Other ______
		☐ Blood ☐ Mucus ☐ Other ______
		☐ Blood ☐ Mucus ☐ Other ______
	More?	

Other Symptoms

- ☐ Bloating
- ☐ Fatigue
- ☐ Nausea
- ☐ Flatulence
- ☐ Vomiting
- ☐ Other ______________________

Stress Level

Sleep

Energy Level

Activity Level

Pain Location (If Applicable)

- ☐ Abdomen
- ☐ Joints
- ☐ Stomach
- ☐ Rectum
- ☐ Other ______________________

Medications

____

____

____

____

____

Notes

Daily Tracking

DATE:

S M T W T F S

Fluid Tracker 8 oz 8 oz 8 oz 8 oz 8 oz 8 oz 8 oz 8 oz

Meal Tracking

Time	Meal	Pain Scale 0-5 0= No pain 5= Severe
BREAKFAST		
LUNCH		
DINNER		
SNACKS		

Bowel Activity

Normal	Very Hard	Abnormalities
		☐ Blood ☐ Mucus ☐ Other ____
		☐ Blood ☐ Mucus ☐ Other ____
		☐ Blood ☐ Mucus ☐ Other ____
		☐ Blood ☐ Mucus ☐ Other ____
	More?	

Other Symptoms

☐ Bloating ☐ Fatigue
☐ Nausea ☐ Flatulence
☐ Vomiting
☐ Other ____________

Stress Level

Sleep

Energy Level

Activity Level

Pain Location (If Applicable)

☐ Abdomen ☐ Joints
☐ Stomach ☐ Rectum
☐ Other ____________

Medications

____
____
____
____
____

Notes

Daily Tracking

DATE:

S M T W T F S

Fluid Tracker: 8 oz | 8 oz | 8 oz | 8 oz | 8 oz | 8 oz | 8 oz | 8 oz

Meal Tracking

Time	Meal	Pain Scale 0-5 0= No pain 5= Severe
BREAKFAST		
LUNCH		
DINNER		
SNACKS		

Bowel Activity

Normal	Very Hard	Abnormalities
		☐ Blood ☐ Mucus ☐ Other ____
		☐ Blood ☐ Mucus ☐ Other ____
		☐ Blood ☐ Mucus ☐ Other ____
		☐ Blood ☐ Mucus ☐ Other ____
	More?	

Other Symptoms

- ☐ Bloating
- ☐ Fatigue
- ☐ Nausea
- ☐ Flatulence
- ☐ Vomiting
- ☐ Other ______________

Stress Level

Sleep

Energy Level

Activity Level

Pain Location (If Applicable)

- ☐ Abdomen
- ☐ Joints
- ☐ Stomach
- ☐ Rectum
- ☐ Other ______________

Medications

____

____

____

____

____

Notes

Daily Tracking

DATE:

S M T W T F S

Fluid Tracker 8 oz 8 oz 8 oz 8 oz 8 oz 8 oz 8 oz 8 oz

Meal Tracking

Time	Meal	Pain Scale 0-5 0= No pain 5= Severe
BREAKFAST		
LUNCH		
DINNER		
SNACKS		

Bowel Activity

Normal	Very Hard	Abnormalities
		☐ Blood ☐ Mucus ☐ Other ____
		☐ Blood ☐ Mucus ☐ Other ____
		☐ Blood ☐ Mucus ☐ Other ____
		☐ Blood ☐ Mucus ☐ Other ____
	More?	

Other Symptoms

☐ Bloating ☐ Fatigue
☐ Nausea ☐ Flatulence
☐ Vomiting
☐ Other ____________________

Stress Level

Sleep

Energy Level

Activity Level

Pain Location (If Applicable)

☐ Abdomen ☐ Joints
☐ Stomach ☐ Rectum
☐ Other ____________________

Medications

____
____
____
____
____

Notes

Weekly Reflections

What was the best thing that happened this week?

What was the hardest thing that happened this week?

What helped you the most this week?

What gave you hope this week?

What's one small win you can celebrate?

Was there something that eased your stress?

Overall, this week I felt

☐ A little better ☐ A lot better ☐ A little worse ☐ A lot worse
☐ About the same

Next week I want to:

____

____

____

____

Healing is often invisible. Trust that small, steady care builds unseen strength.

Monthly Thoughts

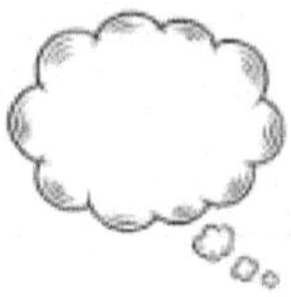

This page is your space to step back and see the bigger picture. Each month brings its own challenges and small victories—use this space to notice patterns, celebrate progress, and reflect on what your body and mind are teaching you. These notes can guide you forward with greater clarity and self-compassion.

This Month I Noticed...

(Write down patterns in your symptoms, energy, or mood.)

Biggest Challenge: ______________________________

____

Brightest Moment: ______________________________

____

Triggers I Noticed: ______________________________

____

Things That Helped: ______________________________

____

Medication / Treatment Notes: (Any changes, side effects, or adjustments.) ______________________________

____

____

Self-Care Check-In

How well I cared for myself this month: ______________________________

____

Looking Forward

Next month I want to focus on: ______________________________

____

____

Symptom Overview

Good Days: ________ Mild Days: ________ Flare Days: ________

Your story is still unfolding, page by page

When You're Feeling...

Your feelings matter. This page gives you space to notice and name your emotions without judgment. Recording them can help you see connections between how you feel and what your body experiences, offering clarity and self-understanding over time.

When I Feel Anxious
It's okay to move slowly—calm often begins with one small step.
Write down three things that feel safe or familiar right now.

When I Feel Discouraged
Even in hard seasons, growth is happening beneath the surface.
What is one small victory you've had recently, even if it feels tiny?

When I Feel Overwhelmed
You don't have to do everything at once—just the next gentle thing.
List three tasks, thoughts, or worries. Circle the one you can focus on first.

When I Feel Hopeful
Hope is the light that reminds you tomorrow can be brighter.
What are three things you're looking forward to, no matter how small?

When I Feel Grateful
Gratitude helps you see what is already good around you.
Write down three people, places, or moments you're thankful for today.

When I Feel Content
Contentment is finding peace in the present moment.
What does 'enough' feel like to you right now? Write a few sentences about it.

Appointment Log

Date	Time	Care Giver	Location

Questions for the Doctor

Notes from the Doctor Visit

Medication and Treatment Notes

Infusions / Injections

Date	Medication/Dosage

Infusions / Injections Cont'd

Date	Medication/Dosage

Steroid Chart

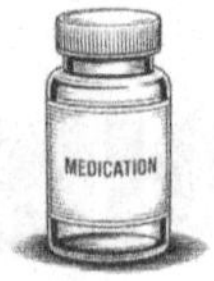

In the event, your doctor prescribes steroids for your treatments, here is a quick chart to help you track them.

Fill in the week (1, 2, 3, etc.) then enter the dosage for that week in the second column (this could change week by week), then enter the number of tablets (optional). Check as you take the medication, put a check mark in the Day column to show that you have taken it. To make it easier, mark out the boxes that you are not using.

Week	Dose	# of tabs	Day 1	Day 2	Day 3	Day 4	Day 5	Day 6	Day 7	Day 8	Day 9	Day 10

In The Hospital

Hospital Name: ____
location: ____
Date Admitted: ____________ Date Released ______________

Physicians

Attending: ___________________ Gastro: _____________________
Surgeon: ____________________ Other: _____________________

Other Medical Personnel

Date	Shift	Name	Role

In The Hospital Cont'd

Procedures / Tests

Date	Procedure

Medications

Date	Medications not listed elsewhere

In The Hospital

Hospital Name: ____________________
location: ____________________
Date Admitted: __________ Date Released __________

Physicians

Attending: __________ Gastro: __________
Surgeon: __________ Other: __________

Other Medical Personnel

Date	Shift	Name	Role

In The Hospital Cont'd

Procedures / Tests

Date	Procedure

Medications

Date	Medications not listed elsewhere

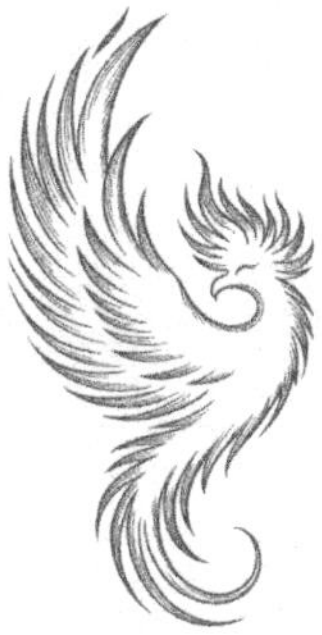

Your Journey Continues

Living with Crohn's or IBD is not a simple path, but it is one we can walk with courage and care. I don't claim to have all the answers—I'm still learning every day. What I do know is that you are stronger than you realize, and that even small steps toward understanding your body matter deeply. remember that your story is still unfolding. The pages you've filled are more than notes they are a testament to your courage, patience, and care for yourself. Every step forward, no matter how small, is part of your healing journey. Carry with you the insights you've discovered here, and let them guide you with compassion and strength.

As you close this journal, I hope you carry forward not only what you've recorded here, but also the knowledge that you are not alone. May your journey ahead be gentler, brighter, and filled with more good days than hard ones.

Made in United States
North Haven, CT
05 November 2026

21765348R00141